THE CHOLESTEROL PUZZLE
THE HORMONE CONNECTION

THE CHOLESTEROL PUZZLE

THE HORMONE CONNECTION

By Jill D. Davey
With Sergey A Dzugan MD PhD

Matador
9 Priory Business Park,
Wistow Road, Kibworth Beauchamp,
Leicestershire. LE8 0RX
Tel: 0116 279 2299
Email: books@troubador.co.uk
Web: www.troubador.co.uk/matador
Twitter: @matadorbooks

ISBN 978 1788033 336

British Library Cataloguing in Publication Data.
A catalogue record for this book is available from the British Library.

Typeset in 11pt Aldine401 BT by Troubador Publishing Ltd, Leicester, UK

Matador is an imprint of Troubador Publishing Ltd

I dedicate this book to my mother, Nora Cambridge Davey, a caring, positive, determined woman, who was always there to listen and to help others. And to William Davey, a witty, generous to a fault, fun-loving, ever-supportive father. Thank you, mum and dad, for making me the person I am today. I miss you with every passing day. To my husband, Giorgio Grassi, the man who is always by my side – a kind, honest, patient and adoring husband; the man who is my safe harbour; to my two sons, Jonathan and Joshua Grassi, who are always there for me, no questions asked; and finally to my dear and lifelong friend Dianne Murray, the girl who encourages and pushes me to the extreme, who protects me and keeps an eye out for me – a friend whom I can truly trust... in every sense of the word. The woman who has helped me to get where I want to be... where I am today and where I am going to go tomorrow. Thank you, Dianne.

Jill D Davey

Dedicated to my grandchildren, Nadya and Misha, for bringing so much enjoyment, love and excitement into my life.

Dr. Dzugan

Jill D Davey is the founder and CEO of www.menopausewoman. com. Jill is an expert in bioidentical hormones therapy and restorative medicine, and is a sought-after speaker in Europe and Asia. Jill is on a mission to inspire and educate women on restorative medicine through her books and coaching.

Sergey A Dzugan MD PhD is co-founder and Chief Scientific Officer of the Dzugan Institute of Restorative Medicine, Deerfield Beach, FL. Dr Dzugan is a former heart surgeon. International Academy of Creative Endeavors (Russia) awarded Dr Dzugan with the honorary title of Academician for outstanding contribution to the development of new methods of hypercholesterolemia and migraine treatment. He performed presentations multiple times at the prestigious International Congress on Anti-Aging Medicine and other medical conferences. He is the author of 157 publications in medical journals, author of seven books, holder of three patents, and author of numerous articles in health-related magazines. Dr Dzugan is a Member of the Editorial Board of the Neuroendocrinology Letters and a Member of the Medical Advisory Board at Life Extension Magazine. He is co-founder and President of iPOMS (International Physiology Optimization Medical Society).

ACKNOWLEDGEMENT

To Dr Sergey Dzugan, who has been instrumental in teaching me the essential and important role that both cholesterol and steroid hormones play in overall health. And how both heart and optimal health can be achieved through bioidentical hormone restorative therapy (BHRT). I call him the 'patient man'! When I ask, he answers... a thousand questions at a time, explaining clearly and precisely how and why things happen within the body. Pinging me over studies and medical articles that I then have to read in-depth, make sense of, and understand. "When you do not understand, you cannot possibly learn. When you do not have the correct information (and the world is full of misinformation), you will never know the truth," he often says. And this is so true. We need to understand, and we so desperately need the information within this book; we need to know the truth – both doctor and layperson alike!

Thank you, Dr Dzugan, for your time and inexhaustible knowledge. I could not have asked for a better teacher. Thank you for taking the time to write this book with me.

To the many doctors, scientists and personalities who have contributed to the advancement of restorative medicine and the use of bioidentical hormones – without you we would not be where we are today. Thank you to each and every one of you.

CONTENTS

FOREWORD BY PHIL MICANS, MS, PHARMB

Cholesterol is an essential substance within our bodies; without it we would be dead in an instant. Yet despite the fact that it remains at the root of all of our hormones, there is a common misconception amongst both the public and even the medical field alike that: 'less is healthier!' That's why this book by Dr Sergey Dzugan and Jill D Davey is such an important read. It helps to set the record straight and explain in a clear and concise way exactly what cholesterol does, what to expect from it and how to manage it correctly, and that doesn't mean with statin drugs!

Thankfully, more and more people are waking up to the pharmaceutical industry's approach, which is essentially marketing their multibillion-dollar statin drugs, and how this blights the real science behind true health and healing.

Thus it falls to the authors of *The Cholesterol Puzzle: The Hormone Connection* to highlight the scientific and clinical benefits of cholesterol; their approach is not masked by the need to make money from product sales, instead they do so in a way that everyone can understand, and it is refreshing to see the facts laid out in an appropriate manner that makes common sense.

If cholesterol is of concern to you, a loved one, a friend, or if your physician has recommended that you take a statin drug to manage your cholesterol, then I strongly advise you read this book.

With this information you will arm yourself with referenced facts, give yourself a 'second opinion' and help yourself make validated judgements that are essential to your long-term health.

Phil Micans, MS, PharmB
Editor, Aging Matters™ Magazine
Assistant Editor, Lifespan Medicine Journal

FOREWORD BY TIM BEAN
AND ANNE LAING

This brilliant book, *The Cholesterol Puzzle: The Hormone Connection*, arms professionals and laymen alike with a personal understanding of their health and how cholesterol has been hijacked as the bad guy in the face of massive research to the contrary. Together, Dr Dzugan and Jill D Davey offer a definitive guide on how to regain control of our health.

If you or a loved one are in the clutches of a statin-pushing physician, this is a great book to delve into and also a great gift to give. Even our own doctor loved it. It opens up a whole new world of truth and logic that will empower everyone – you, your friend, your relative – to start taking control of their own health and rethink the current destructive paradigm that often exists on the other side of the waiting room.

Tim Bean and Anne Laing, Co-Owners/Directors at
Performance Training Company, New Zealand.

INTRODUCTION

Did you ever get the feeling that something was not quite right, that there was a lot more to the cholesterol story than you were being told? Well, your instincts served you well. There is… a lot more! For decades we have been led to believe that elevated cholesterol levels in the blood are dangerous and lead to heart attack, stroke, and even death. This thought pattern is now obsolete. And for decades we have been led to believe that the best way to deal with high cholesterol and avoid a heart attack is to ingest a cholesterol-lowering drug. This thought pattern is now also obsolete. Truth be known, low levels of cholesterol are just as detrimental to your health, if not more so. What is really needed, and is now considered the 'modern approach' or 'new thought pattern', is a normalized level of cholesterol (which equates to neither too high nor too low a level), which in turn will take you to the realms of optimal health and protect you against heart disease. How to achieve this is all explained within the pages of this book.

At this point we should be asking ourselves, what really does cause cardiovascular disease? And could the health of our heart really be solely dependent on one single marker such as total cholesterol levels and one simplistic solution such as a statin drug? No! The body is a little more complex than that.

Cardiovascular disease is still the number-one killer in the Western world even when there is an abundance of statins on the marketplace. Cholesterol-lowering drugs such as statins inhibit cholesterol production, therefore, lower it. If statins were doing the job they were designed to do (reduce heart-attack events by lowering cholesterol), and if cholesterol were really the true culprit behind the occurrence of a heart attack, then surely there should have been a significant reduction in heart-attack events, but there hasn't! So something is wrong; it doesn't make sense. And, if we take a look at various studies, we can see that almost 50% of people who have had heart attacks do not have high cholesterol levels. Again, it doesn't make sense. Is it not the build-up of cholesterol in the artery walls that provokes a heart attack? Reviewing these facts and many more that are contained within this book, it seems that conventional medicine has hit a concrete wall when it comes to reducing and treating this issue appropriately.

However, this book is not intended to be yet another 'cholesterol/statin' episode, telling you more of the same thing. It is so much more than that. This book is different. This book offers you cutting-edge technology for the correction of cholesterol disorders and, at the same time, holds the key to obtaining optimal health. This book discusses a totally different viewpoint of why and how cholesterol levels increase with age and the interconnection with steroid-hormone synthesis. This book offers you a whole new way of looking at medicine.

This book is revolutionary! This book offers you a natural, safe and efficient solution for the restoration of normal cholesterol metabolism and the treatment and prevention of heart disease, together with the possibility of perfect health interwoven with positive longevity without the use of any chemical drugs, including statins. This book offers you life! It offers you the truth and a new beginning. This book tells you how to overcome hypercholesterolemia, not by taking a statin drug, or by diet, or with exercise, but with the use of restorative medicine which in turn will help you to live a high-quality, long and disease-free life at 360 degrees.

Restorative medicine is breakthrough medicine that offers a new and different approach to health. It is a medicine that works, a medicine that is safe, effective and natural. It is a medicine that is aimed at early detection, prevention, treatment and reversal of age-related dysfunction, disorders and diseases, in both men and women. It is a medicine that tips the 'seesaw' in your favor by correcting hormonal deficiencies that naturally occur with age. The correcting of hormone deficiencies will, in turn, correct the age-related metabolic shift from catabolic (breakdown/damage) to anabolic (repair/build) process, helping to protect against tissue degeneration, including that of the heart.

This book explains that high cholesterol levels are not, in fact, the primary cause or indicator of heart disease but, instead, are a marker that something is dysfunctioning in the body. It explains that coronary heart disease does not occur because of cholesterol but because of an initial injury or microtrauma to the endothelium (the innermost layer of the arteries), which is caused by many different factors such as cigarette smoke, high levels of sugar (glucose) in the blood, 'wear and tear' on the arterial walls, toxins, oxidized LDL, heavy metals, and elevated blood pressure. Cholesterol is a repair molecule and is found in the arteries for that reason: it is there to repair the damage or microtrauma; it is not there to deliberately clog up the arteries.

In this book, Dr Dzugan and I explain the real truth behind hypercholesterolemia and coronary heart disease, how to treat it, prevent it and, importantly, how to resolve it naturally. This book gives you a new angle on the word 'cholesterol'. It explains how the heart functions and what really does cause heart disease. It shows in detail the numerous side effects (deleterious or otherwise) statins cause and, importantly, why they occur because of these drugs. It presents a reason why doctors should think 'ten times' before prescribing these drugs and why patients should think 'twenty times' before taking them. It explains why both doctor and patient should be moving towards restorative medicine and embracing the revolutionary hypothesis presented by Dr Dzugan in this book – a dynamic hypothesis that corrects the issue of hypercholesterolemia and, again, we emphasize, without the use of any chemical drugs, including statins. This is known as the hormonodeficit hypothesis and it will be fully explained within the pages of this book, in an easy, step-by-step guide. This hypothesis is your answer, your way out.

This book leads to understanding and gives you all the relevant information needed to enable you to make an informed decision about your heart health and your health in general. This book is your health and heart problem solver! This book will save your life. It can save you from 'death by a statin'. What is it they say? 'Information is power!' This book is powerful information.

If someone were to tell you that cholesterol-lowering drugs did not, in fact, save you from heart attack and that they actually increased your risk of stroke, of a devastating type, caused by bleeding into the brain, would you consider taking these drugs? And what if someone were to tell you that cholesterol is far from the villain in your life and that, instead, it is a vital part of every cell in the body? And what if someone were to tell you that cholesterol plays many important functions in the body and is the most abundantly produced molecule in the human body, and is produced in such high quantities because it is important for normally functioning physiology? In other words, cholesterol is part of the human machinery and networking systems that enable the body to function correctly. If someone were to tell you all of this, together with even more disturbing information, would you still consider or continue taking a statin drug or would you look towards a natural, safe and efficient method of correcting hypercholesterolemia – a method that lies within the pages of this book?

One of cholesterol's major functions is to act as the building block for the manufacture of steroid hormones, including sex hormones such as estrogens, progesterone and testosterone. Again, the mechanism of the statin drug is to inhibit cholesterol production, which will therefore interfere and decrease hormone production. Hormones are not only there for reproductive purposes, they are, in fact, the most significant messaging machine in the human body. They are what Dr Dzugan and I consider to be 'The Human Network of Health'. Hormones are the most independent factor for a healthy, strong and vibrant immune system.

They are the main molecule in regeneration and repair: they build us up or tear us down. They dictate who we are, our health, our strength, our power, our emotions, our sensuality, our very being. From the moment we are born they dictate how we develop, grow, age, and how we die. What are we going to do without cholesterol and, therefore, hormones, for that matter? We are certainly not going to stay healthy for long and we will certainly die at an earlier age due to this deficiency. That is perhaps why individuals on cholesterol-lowering drugs are at a higher risk of death from all causes, including cancer.

This book explains why cholesterol levels increase with age and why steroid hormones decline with age. Cholesterol is the precursor of steroid hormones and, with age, hormones decline. Because of this decline, cholesterol production increases, to try and compensate for this slack in hormone production but, as the systems in place for adequate hormone production also break down as we age, cholesterol levels remain and will remain elevated, unless some intervention takes place. This is where Dr Dzugan's hypothesis fits in. This is where the missing piece of the puzzle of lipid disorders clicks perfectly into place. Dr Dzugan did it. This unique and extraordinary approach to such a complex issue allows for the optimization of body physiology that then leads to the full restoration of a normal cholesterol metabolism. No more high cholesterol!

This is information that you will not get from your doctor; he or she most likely doesn't know anything about it (no disrespect meant). This information is vital for your health and for your life. You deserve to have this information! You deserve to have a solution to heart disease and optimal overall health. It is your right.

How It All Started: The Initiation of The Hormonodeficit Hypothesis

As a former heart surgeon, Dr Dzugan often posed the question to himself: why was it that so many individuals who'd had heart attacks had normal cholesterol levels? Whenever a biological malfunction occurs, the next logical step, in his opinion, is to find the scientific explanation behind this event. The next thread to this hypothesis came about when Dr Dzugan was working at the North Central Regional Cancer Center in Greenwood, Mississippi, USA, together with Dr Arnold Smith, where immunorestorative therapy is used for cancer patients. The core element of immunorestorative therapy is hormonorestorative therapy. Simply put, when hormone levels are restored, in large part the immune system is also restored. One of these experiences made an impressive mark on Dr Dzugan, one which turned into a very strong idea.

One particular patient had advanced non-small-cell lung cancer. He had an inoperable tumor with multiple metastases that had spread to the brain, chest and lymph nodes in the neck. He underwent radiation treatment and then was given immunorestorative therapy. For many years, he'd had a cholesterol level that was considered high by conventional medicine – 300 mg/dL – was on statin drugs and took a large dose of insulin due to his insulin-dependent diabetes. After his immunorestorative therapy, his cholesterol levels were tested, which revealed that his levels had normalized (without the use of statin drugs, as they were stopped before cancer treatment). This started Dr Dzugan thinking and he shortly realized that this patient was not the only one whose cholesterol levels had normalized after immunorestorative therapy.

This is when Dr Dzugan decided to review the pathway of cholesterol metabolism. What he found was somewhat more than interesting. He found that hormone production decreased with age, while cholesterol production increased. This increase was due to a feedback loop mechanism, which is simply explained in this book.

This was the turning of the key, the opening of the door to a new beginning, to a new cholesterol story that clearly provides the evidence, eliminating all the negative information that is currently and consistently attacking both doctors and laypeople.

This is the beginning of a new cholesterol story. This time it is the *right* story, the *correct* story, the *true* story! Everything is in place; no doubts or question marks are hanging around that need to be answered. Everything is clearly and logically explained in this book. Everything makes sense.

1. THE TRUTH ABOUT CHOLESTEROL AND THE STATIN DISASTER

Cholesterol – what and who took us to where we are today? And how did we get into this state? Cholesterol – why is it we are so afraid of this life-giving molecule? Simple word, complex situation. Cholesterol – heart attack. What, how and when did this mixed-up notion of cholesterol and its connection to the world's number-one killer, heart disease, begin?

Why is it that nearly everyone at age fifty plus either takes or is advised to take a cholesterol-lowering drug (CLD), statins being the best known? If we backtrack, it is crystal clear that it began when conventional medicine focused on cholesterol as the supposed culprit of atherosclerosis (plaque in the arteries) over half a century ago. Statins are a multibillion-dollar business; it's what we like to call a 'push' business. It seems that, even with an abundance of CLDs on the marketplace, conventional medicine has hit a concrete wall when it comes to reducing and treating cardiovascular disease appropriately. To understand why, we need to look at science, in the true sense of the word. Restorative medicine is based on solid scientific research and evidence. With that said, let's first take a look at the real cause of atherosclerosis and arteriosclerosis (hardening of the arteries).

A Brief Look at Heart Disease

Heart disease is a term generally used to identify a number of diseases, of which there are many, that affect the heart and sometimes the blood vessels. Heart disease or cardiovascular disease (CVD) include: coronary artery disease (CAD), arrhythmias (irregular heart beat), blocked vessels (that may lead to insufficient blood circulation or stroke), heart infections and heart defects we are born with, and acquired valve damages.

To a layperson like myself, heart disease would appear to mean 'a disease of the heart', but atherosclerosis, the subject which Dr Dzugan and I are about to talk of, is not actually a disease of the heart but a disease of the arteries that supply blood to the heart.

Simply put, the cardiovascular system consists of a heart that pumps the blood and the blood vessels that carry blood to all parts of the body and then return it to the heart. The blood vessels that carry blood away from the heart are called arteries, while veins carry blood towards the heart. It is the arteries that we are interested in when we talk about cardiovascular disease.

Arteries are complex, and a multilayered living tube. We generally think of the arteries as transporting oxygenated blood from the heart to all parts of the body, but they have other important tasks to do as well. As an example, they ensure that the blood flow is kept at the right speed and physical consistency. When the arteries dysfunction, the end result can be lethal.

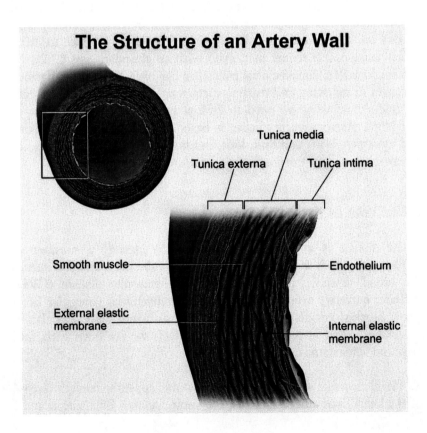

The Structure of an Artery Wall

Tunica media

Tunica externa

Tunica intima

Smooth muscle

Endothelium

External elastic membrane

Internal elastic membrane

The central part of the artery is called the lumen: this is the open area – somewhat like a corridor, let's say – where the blood flows through. The blood travels through this corridor along with red blood cells, white blood cells, proteins, nutrients, platelets, oxygen and other substances. The layer in which the blood actually makes contact is called the intima. The intima is made up of a smooth inner lining, plus connective tissue, and is known as the endothelium. Moving further into the arterial wall we get to the media, which is a thicker layer made up of smooth muscle. The outermost layer is called the adventitia and is mainly made up of connective tissue which helps support the artery, preventing it from bulging outwards.

The arteries are far from being an inert pipe or a solid, ridged highway for the blood to run through; instead, they are like an accommodating musical instrument (composed of smooth muscle, media) that contracts in response to the rhythm of the heart and the pulsing of the blood. Arteries are a very dynamic and vital organ that is, in essence, a living, breathing part of our body. The endothelium is the 'starting area' in which coronary heart disease begins. The endothelium is only one cell thick but is where an incredible amount of biochemical activity occurs. There are more than 400 biochemical and biomechanical mediators of endothelial dysfunction, meaning, things that can harm the endothelium. It is the main protective barrier that defends the artery against harmful agents that can travel in the blood, agents such as nicotine, sugar, oxidized LDL (low-density lipoprotein) and toxins. The name 'endothelium dysfunction' is used to describe a pathological state where damage to the innermost layer exists. The endothelium not only acts as a barrier, it also has other tasks, including fighting off disease by regulating the way the immune system behaves within the arteries, protecting against bacteria and other invaders or pathogens. It regulates blood pressure and arterial tone, it controls oxidative stress – a process by which cells, tissues, organs and bodily systems, including and in particular the cardiovascular system, become damaged due to an imbalance between the production of free radicals (unstable molecules responsible for the aforementioned damage and the ability of the body to counteract or detoxify their harmful effects by way of neutralization with antioxidants) and inflammation, and maintains homeostasis (balance) by way of detecting and responding to changes in blood content (e.g. oxygen) and status. It helps keep the blood thin and fluid enough so that it can flow through the vessels easily, and it controls blood-clotting. As you will have understood, the endothelium is so much more than just a motionless tube, it is the 'brainpower' of the arteries, protecting us from toxins, bacteria and other agents that can either harm or change its function and behavior. When the innermost layer is damaged, the pathway is to heart disease.

Today, it is common belief that heart disease begins with atherosclerosis (clogging of the arteries) because of an excess or high amount of cholesterol flowing in the bloodstream which then sticks to the inner lining of the arteries. This school of thought is now obsolete. We now know that heart disease begins with an injury or lesion to the endothelium. Think of this injury as something like a 'microscopic scratch', something so small you can hardly see it. As Dr Dzugan explained to me, "Heart disease begins because of an injury to the endothelium. Atherosclerosis is a physiological adaptation to vascular damage or injury, and is part of a failed healing process." First comes the damage or injury to the tissue, then comes an accumulation of various powerful healing materials such as cholesterol, and then a scar-like tissue forms. This is part of the healing process of the wound from the damage that has taken place. As stated previously, many things can cause this damage (more than 400), including cigarette smoke, toxins, heavy metals, oxidized LDL cholesterol, general 'wear and tear' on the arterial walls, elevated blood pressure, and high levels of blood sugar (glucose) as seen in diabetics, to name a few.

A Quick Note about How Sugar Can Directly Affect the Heart

Excess sugar in the diet or bloodstream is not good and can directly affect the heart. A continual excess of sugar in the bloodstream will bring an increase of insulin (a hormone produced by the pancreas which helps shuttle excess sugar out of the bloodstream into the cells). This in turn can provoke insulin resistance which will eventually provoke diabetes type 2. When there is a continual overload of sugar in the bloodstream, the pancreas will get to the point where it can no longer cope with the added demand for more and more insulin, even though the cells may still be able to absorb sufficient sugar to stop you from becoming truly diabetic.

It is interesting to note that, with age, glucose levels often elevate. In our opinion, this is due to the fact that the cells require the same amount of glucose they had in our younger years; however, the sensitivity of the cell membrane becomes significantly worse during the aging process. This means that the cells are unable to absorb a sufficient amount of glucose required for optimal function, leaving an excess in the bloodstream. The cells require but the body doesn't need this excess, or larger concentration, of glucose in the blood. It is the *cells* that demand an excess of glucose in the bloodstream, as they are trying to keep the same level of glucose as in their younger years.

When there is an excess of sugar floating around, we are in a bad situation. The endothelium is made up of cells that line the inside of the blood vessels; these cells secrete nitric oxide which, when secreted in the correct quantities, keeps the blood vessels open. When we consume an excess amount of sugar, it enters the endothelium cells and will cause them to dysfunction. The endothelium then secretes less nitric oxide, giving way to high blood pressure – high blood pressure damages the arteries! When the correct amount of nitric oxide is secreted, you will have the correct blood pressure, good circulation in general and, for you men, good erectile function. Sound good?

The arteries of the heart and the rest of the body have very small muscles built into their walls which control the dilation and contraction of the arteries. When these muscles contract, they narrow the diameter of the arteries and, when they relax, the arteries open up again. It is the nervous system that controls the flow of blood to the arteries and takes on the task of increasing or decreasing it, as appropriate. In medical terms, this is called 'arterial compliance'; in layman's terms, this is called the 'push-and-flow mechanism' (that's how I see it, anyway). We should remember that the arteries contract and relax twenty-four hours a day against the force of the blood, they are never at peace. They must maintain their functional and structural integrity to keep us safe. Generally, the health of the muscles in the arteries is supported by anabolic (building) hormones, which significantly decrease with age. When anabolic hormones decline, so too does the support mechanism that protects these muscles. When the endothelium is damaged and therefore compromised, and the muscles become weaker due to an anabolic hormonal decline, it cannot function as it should. Blood traveling at the correct speed and manner is not a problem but, when there are alterations in this speed or manner, it will raise the risk of heart disease largely by damaging the endothelium. Any insult or damage to the endothelium raises the risk of heart disease.

Heart disease is the number-one killer, in both men and women, worldwide.

Q: But which form of heart disease?
A: Atherosclerosis.

'Athero' or 'atheroma' is used to describe a build-up of fatty, grey goo or gunk that forms in the artery walls. 'Sclerosis', on the other hand, means thickening or hardening. *Et voilà!* We now have a very dangerous scenario: atherosclerosis. These thickenings are sometimes called atherosclerotic or atheromatous plaque or, more simply, plaque. An accumulation of plaque in the arteries will eventually cause the vessels to narrow or to become completely blocked. When this happens, oxygen and nutrients carried by the blood will be unable to reach the heart. When the heart is not receiving the amount of blood it needs, it is described as being 'ischemic', hence the term 'ischemic heart disease' (IHD), also known as coronary heart disease (CHD).

Common Risk Factors for Heart Disease

Age is the most powerful risk factor of cardiovascular disease. Menopause and andropause, which mark the end of normal gonadal function, increase cardiovascular-disease risk because of the age-related decline in sex hormones. It is these hormones that give us a natural protection against coronary heart disease. Men are usually more prone to developing heart disease than women, at least until after menopause when a woman's risk then becomes the same as a man's. Coronary heart disease rarely occurs prior to these age-related changes. Diabetes, diet, genetics, stress, lack of exercise, high blood pressure (hypertension), obesity and hygiene (poor hygiene can lead to infections which increase the risk of developing heart disease) are other risk factors.

Underlying Factors Involved in Atherosclerosis

Excess triglycerides, low blood EPA/DHA (Omega-3s), elevated C-reactive Protein, oxidized LDL particles, high glucose, nitric-oxide deficit, low vitamin K, excess insulin, hypertension, excess fibrinogen (clot-promoting substance), excess homocysteine, low testosterone, excess cholesterol... Over a lifetime, the aging human suffers microscopic trauma or tiny pinpricks of the arteries from these various assaults, the cumulative effect being a build-up of plaque (arterial occlusion) which can provoke angina or an acute heart attack.

Understanding Plaque Build-up

The initial microscopic erosion or pinprick on the endothelium will set off a chain reaction, which is classed as inflammation, rushing white blood cells, platelets and other immune cells to patch things up. This type of inflammation is known as aseptic inflammation, meaning, it has no association with infection, rather, it is damage-associated inflammation. Without this damage, the inflammation process will not be initiated. The body sees this vascular microtrauma as a threat and needs to get rid of it by way of repair, by healing the damage and correcting the underlying problem. The only thing is, these immune cells don't just rush over and seal up the lesion with some kind of molecular liquid repair kit and say "'that's that all fixed then'" and go home. Instead, some cells bind to the site of damage, while others actually chew ('chew' because they are trying to destroy the invader and protect the body) their way through the endothelium and into the artery walls, which in turn will alter endothelium function and initiate heart disease.

Basically, the immune system perceives the microtrauma as a threat so sends in the recruited army in an attempt to isolate or seal off the injured or damaged area, to remove it, and then to begin the process of healing the damage that has occurred. It is our immune system that protects us from pathogens and the 'invader'. It is the initial damage done by the various components to the endothelium that sets the stage for this scene – heart disease.

A Quick Look at This Scene

Monocytes (the largest of the white blood cells which ingest large foreign particles and cell debris) are ready to ambush this foreign object, scurry to the scene and release chemicals called cytokines (these are essentially chemical messengers that help regulate the immune-system response). Unfortunately, though, many of these cytokines are highly inflammatory and will go on to cause the endothelium to produce glue-like molecules called adhesion molecules or adhesins. These glue-like molecules then capture the monocytes that initially came to halt these foreign invaders. These monocytes now change into macrophages. Macrophages are actually large white blood cells, large because of their function. The Greek translation for macrophage literally means 'large and eat' and that's what they do: they guzzle up the enemy; they are helpful immune-system cells in the true sense of the word. Any molecular rubbish (toxins, etc.) is engulfed by these large white blood cells. Macrophages specifically contribute to plaque, in fact, they are the largest component of atherosclerotic plaque, but are also extremely vital to the regular function of the body, protecting on their travels.

These immune-system cells – along with cholesterol, smooth-muscle cells, inflammatory cells, cytokines and clotting substances such as fibrin and platelets – will eventually combine to form a toxic, yucky gunk within the inner artery walls. Once the toxic brew has formed, the body will create a thin fortress as a safety mechanism to try and wall it off; this is what is known as 'unstable' or 'vulnerable' plaque. But all is not safe. The toxic poison will attract even more immune-system cells, turning the once helpful macrophages into harmful foam cells, which keeps the process going. Over time, the poisonous brew

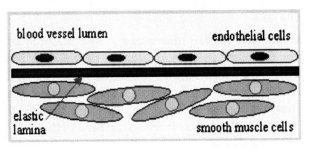

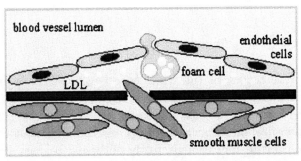

inside the artery walls grows larger and more dangerous, and becomes covered with a fibrous cap – a kind of scab, if you like. Eventually, once the build-up has become advanced enough, calcification occurs, causing the outer edges to become inelastic, harder and stiffer, thus narrowing the arteries. This is a condition known as arteriosclerosis.

The danger with unstable or vulnerable plaque is that the scab may come off or rupture. If this yucky, gooey mess that is inside the thin-walled fortress makes contact with the blood flowing through the artery (bloodstream), another chain reaction immediately takes place. An extremely powerful message is sent to the blood-clotting system to try and seal off this rupture. The result is a blood clot (also known as thrombus), which then forms over the burst plaque. A blood clot is effectively the body's way of protecting itself; it's a protective mechanism. If the blood clot is large enough, the blood flow through that artery can be completely interrupted. Therefore, whichever organ is being supplied with the blood will be starved of oxygen and, of course, blood. If the organ is the heart, it may then undergo an 'infarct' – in layman's terms, a 'heart attack'. Heart-muscle damage, caused by an interruption of the blood supply, is called a myocardial infarction (MI) – again, a heart attack.

Infarctions in the Body

A little more information about 'infarctions': apart from the heart, infarctions can happen elsewhere in the body. Large plaques can sometimes form in the carotid arteries (neck). This is definitely not a good place to have plaque (neck/brain connection) as the carotid arteries supply blood to the brain. How it works: a clot forms over the carotid plaque; in the majority of cases, though, the carotid arteries never become totally blocked. What happens is that a part of the clot that has formed over the carotid plaque breaks off and travels to the brain, through even smaller arteries. When the clot reaches a point that is too narrow to pass through, it gets blocked, which effectively dams up the blood supply to an area of the brain, which in turn leads to the most common type of stroke: ischemic stroke, known as cerebral infarction. Another type of stroke that is not considered an infarction is a cerebral hemorrhage (hemorrhagic stroke). It happens when an artery in the brain bursts, causing bleeding into the brain. This is the most devastating type of stroke.

Infarctions can also happen in the kidneys, pelvis, gut, the legs and arms (usually named gangrene) and even the eyes. The aorta, which is the major blood vessel that leads out of the heart down into the chest and abdomen, is another place where infarction may occur. Sounds bad. It is bad.

The Calcium Connection

Along with macrophages, calcium is also found in the build-up of plaque. This calcification will make the heart less responsive to the demands of the body and, of course, harder and stiffer arteries will make it much more difficult to disperse a blockage when need be.

We have to ponder here why is it, then, that older individuals are encouraged to supplement with such high doses of calcium, more so women who are advised to ingest them on a regular basis? Yes, we realize that calcium is good for osteoporosis (along with vitamin D3, since calcium cannot integrate into the bones without sufficient vitamin D3 and magnesium), but there are always two sides to a story. When there is over-supplementation or an excess of calcium in the body, it can increase risk of blood-pressure elevation, arrhythmia, induce sleep problems, constipation and kidney stones. Coronary artery calcification has been well known as an important culprit in heart disease for a long time. But, unfortunately, this obsession with cholesterol is still the major focus. Calcium is good for bones but, when there is an excess of it floating around, it is not good.

Taking a deeper look at calcium: calcium and magnesium have an interesting relationship. Magnesium is a natural calcium blocker, so important in heart health. It has the ability to block the channels by which calcium enters the cells; when magnesium is low, intracellular calcium rises. Magnesium also inhibits platelet accumulation. Platelets, also known as thrombocytes, are cell fragments that circulate in the blood and are responsible for clotting, and are also another component of plaque. We tend to think of platelets as being life-saving particles that prevent us from bleeding to death but, again, there are always two sides to a story. When platelet levels are not optimal, it's not good. Levels that are too low increase the risk of excessive bleeding, whereas levels that are too high increase the risk of blood-clot formation, which can lead to strokes and heart attacks. Perhaps we should consider supplementing with magnesium rather than calcium.

Magnesium also helps lower blood pressure. Magnesium has a relaxing effect on the body, therefore, on the arteries as well. Relaxed arteries allow the blood to flow more easily, putting the heart under less stress. When arteries are narrow and constricted, this dangerously raises blood pressure. When arteries are widened and relaxed, the heart doesn't need to pump or work as much to get the blood through, so blood pressure doesn't rise.

Magnesium also helps regulate blood sugar. Remember, continual high blood sugar will lead to insulin resistance, which will provoke diabetes type 2. Diabetics are on the fast track to heart disease as an overproduction of insulin leads to high blood pressure and hardening of the arteries, as well as free radical (an unstable molecule that causes cell damage) activity, followed by accelerated aging and the development of disease.

Understanding Inflammation

Here's how inflammation works in the body: inflammation is a natural process, it is our safety mechanism. It is a natural defense response in the body to protect against injury, toxins and infections. But inflammation can work for or against us, transitioning from acute to chronic. Inflammation is not just a cut on your finger that turns red, swells and feels hot, or a temperature you have in your body due to an infection. There is more to inflammation than meets the eye. This kind of inflammation is the body working at its most basic level. This is called acute inflammation and is transitory. Our defense mechanism is set to immediately attack any lethal microbes that enter our body; this is the body's way of healing. The body needs a certain amount of inflammation to be healthy. If we do not have it, we cannot fight off infections and kill cancers, for instance. Inflammation is our body at work; it's an indication that pro-inflammatory chemicals in the blood are at work, disabling and healing tissue by way of repair. Inflammation is also linked to aging and declining hormone levels. Age and declining hormones are interrelated. The definition of declining hormones is a hormonal imbalance. Declining hormones bring with them an inability to turn off inflammatory reactions, which creates an imbalance between destructive and protective inflammatory responses. This imbalance creates low-level systemic inflammation that slowly destroys tissue by launching an attack on our normal cells. Our body is gradually shifting into a state of chronic inflammation, also known as inflammaging. Inflammation has now become the chronic form rather than the transitory (acute) form which is needed for our protection. You may not be able to see it but it is there, lurking inside the body. Inflammation, in actual fact, is the body's way of talking to us; it is a message, a warning sign that all is not well within the body.

Chronic inflammation is something deep-rooted. It is not good. It is dangerous. It is age-related, can be genetically related (but this does not mean we have to flick the switch of inflammation) or it can be related to the environment. If we insist on eating badly (an unhealthy diet full of bad fats: a high glycemic diet), smoking, together with no exercise, this puts extra pressure on our body, which keeps the inflammatory process chugging along. Smoking is one of the factors that leads to plaque in the arteries, together with other health problems. Plaque promotes heart disease, which is one definition of chronic inflammation. Apart from cardiovascular disease, chronic inflammation is also linked to conditions such as diabetes, cancers, rheumatoid arthritis, colitis, Alzheimer's, and digestive-system diseases. Chronic inflammation attacks cells throughout the body, causing damage to brain cells and the lining of our arteries, while about 25% of all cancers are linked to chronic inflammation. Chronic inflammation harms us and is associated with nearly every age-related disease there is.

To Cut the Atherosclerosis Story Short

Atherosclerosis is a disease primarily involving four cell types: endothelial, vascular smooth-muscle cells, monocytes and platelets. Arterial plaque contains a complex mixture of cholesterol, calcium, lipoproteins, mutated arterial cells and fibrin. It is well known that the composition of the atheroma is the same as for many granulation tissues which are interpreted as a healing process. Cholesterol is an important process of normal repair of tissue – and not just a substance that is, by default, content on clogging the arteries – as every cell membrane and organelle within the cells is rich in cholesterol (we will discuss cholesterol and its function in the body in the following chapters).

Cholesterol is present along with fibrin, collagen and elastin as part of the repair process to the lesions (initial microscopic scratches). Fibrins, in conjunction with platelets, work to clog the wounds. Collagen and elastin are types of connective tissue. Arterial plaque begins in the form of mutations to smooth-muscle cells in the arteries, which can then proliferate and become fibrous and even create their own cholesterol. The key point to remember and understand is that cholesterol does not start the process of atherosclerosis, rather, it is the end product of degeneration. This is a 'dot-to-dot' situation, but the dots will all join together as you read.

2. CHOLESTEROL CLARITY AND A BRIEF ENCOUNTER WITH STATINS

Cholesterol-Lowering Drugs (CLD)

Cholesterol has been associated with atherosclerosis, the key word being 'associated'. 'Association' is a big word in the statin industry (remember, statins are the most well-known of CLDs) but it is this association that has brought us to where we are today. There is never any mention of what cholesterol does, how it functions within the body and why it is there or, for that matter, why it increases with age. Watch those dots join up…! The mechanism behind statins is to lower cholesterol, today even more so than ever before. The ever-changing levels of cholesterol! Over the years, the 'recommended' cholesterol levels have changed consistently. We are asking, why? Is a level not a level? Do we humans change so dramatically and continually, do our cholesterol levels fluctuate so drastically year in, year out that the pharmaceutical industries are obliged to adjust these levels accordingly or to an ever-decreasing baseline?

There is much controversy about these drugs but we are still stuck in 'stuck mode'. We cannot get away from the fact that cholesterol should be lowered because it is dangerous to the heart. That is the final solution.

'Cholesterol-lowering drugs' (CLD) is a blanket term for various medications but 'statin' is the best-known name. Lipitor (Atorvastatin), Pravachol (Pravastatin), Crestor (Rosuvastatin), Mevacor (Lovastatin – not licensed for use in the UK), Zocor (Simvastatin), and Lescol and Lescol XL (Fluvastatin) are all statins (also known as HMG-CoA reductase inhibitors). Along with statins, there are other CLD groups which come under the names of selective cholesterol absorption inhibitors, resins (bile acid-binding drugs), fibrates, niacin, and proprotein-convertase-subtilisin-kexin-9 (PCSK9) inhibitors. These groups of agents all follow the same theme, affecting the basic mechanism of cholesterol in a major way.

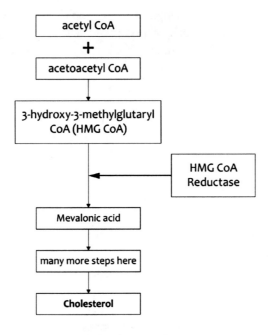

Cholesterol Biosynthesis
(simplified version)

The Mechanism behind How Statins Inhibit Cholesterol

A molecule of cholesterol is primarily synthesized or produced from Acetyl CoA through the reductase pathway known as 3-hydroxy-3-methylglutaryl CoA (HMG-CoA). HMG-CoA is then acted upon by an enzyme called HMG-CoA reductase, which eventually goes on to create the final product: cholesterol. Statins work by inhibiting the enzyme HMG-CoA reductase, therefore cutting off cholesterol production, the raw material, in its prime.

Getting to Know Cholesterol: What Is It?

Cholesterol – simple word but not such a simple molecule. To answer the above question succinctly – cholesterol is one of the most important and most generous molecules in the human body – without it, we could not evolve. To answer it in a more in-depth manner, let's take a look at how cholesterol functions within the body.

Cholesterol has many, many important functions in the body. Cholesterol is a necessary building block of just about every system in the body. In actual fact, to build and maintain a healthy human being, the body requires a hell of a lot of this magnificent substance. So much so that cholesterol is found in all cells of the body, and all cells need cholesterol in their membranes; without it, they would/could not survive; they would kind of just... 'disintegrate'. It is the high amount of cholesterol found in these cell membranes that helps maintain their integrity and also facilitates cellular communication. Cell membranes cover the cells and protect them, acting as a sort of barrier. They are semi-permeable but need to be resistant enough to keep all kinds of molecular 'undesirable trash' out, yet pliable and soft enough to allow 'essential and desirable' molecules in. Cholesterol is needed for optimal function.

Cholesterol is particularly important in the brain, the nervous system, the spinal cord and the peripheral nerves. Without cholesterol, cells wouldn't be able to protect themselves from oxidation, which potentially creates a dangerous scenario. Cholesterol is also an important factor in stabilizing cells against temperature changes. It is vital for the routine repair of tissues and is what gives the skin its ability to shed water.

Cholesterol is so important that 25%, that is, a quarter of all the cholesterol produced in the body, is localized in the brain, with most of it being present in the myelin. Looking at it this way, the brain is 2% of our body weight but contains 25% of our cholesterol. It seems incredible, doesn't it? When we go to sleep at night, the brain produces more cholesterol. What is it, 'Darth Vader' attacking our brain while we sleep? Don't think so! All cholesterol in the brain is a product of local synthesis as plasma lipoproteins are too big to pass or cross the blood-brain barrier. The blood-brain barrier (BBB) is quite simply a division between the blood circulating in our bodies and the fluid surrounding our brain. It is the brain's safeguard. It keeps the invader out, such as bacteria and large molecules, but, at the same time, allows in such things as oxygen and hormones that are required by the brain.

Cholesterol plays a significant role in brain function, especially in the mechanisms of synaptic function, plasticity and neurodegeneration. Central neurodegeneration features in a number of neurodegenerative diseases and may represent functional consequences of abnormal neural cholesterol misregulation.

It seems strange that the brain, our most intelligent organ and a most vital part of the body, should be so rich in cholesterol when it is apparently so dangerous to the human body. Think about that one for a second, please. In essence, all cholesterol in the brain is made in the brain because of this barrier. What's even more interesting is that cholesterol is embedded in the myelin sheath. The myelin sheath is a fatty material made up of 27% cholesterol, 43% phospholipid and 30% protein, which winds around the nerve cell axons. Therefore, basically, the myelin insulates nerve cells, helps regenerate cut axons and intensifies impulses or electrical signals (messages) throughout the nervous system's circuitry. Neuronal communication is not only dependent on cholesterol, it is vital. One in every ten cells in the brain is a neuron. Neurons are the workmen of the brain; they are helping me in my research for this book, for example, helping me to store memory, make memory, tap the keys of my computer, move my arms up and down, stand up and sit down. The other nine-tenths of the cells are known as supportive cells. These supportive cells provide support and protection for neurons in the brain and peripheral nervous system; they repair tissue, repair the neurons, feed nutrients to the neurons and can even generate their own hormones which are known as neurosteroids. As we age, our neurons age and then die, our brain shrinks and cognitive ability declines.

What do you think happens to the brain when cholesterol levels are low? I'll give you a hint. Many degenerative diseases are associated with an imbalance of cholesterol in the brain, including Alzheimer's disease. And that's just for starters! The statin drugs atorvastatin, lovastatin and simvastatin are much more lipophilic (meaning they dissolve in fat) than the others, so they are far more capable of crossing the blood-brain barrier, therefore promoting central-nervous-system disturbances. The others are more hydrophilic (meaning they dissolve in water), therefore much less likely to affect the brain.

Cholesterol is the backbone of every single neurosteroid in the brain. We cannot make neurosteroids without cholesterol. Neurosteroids are important for communication, brain repair and regeneration, the growth of new neurons and the structural maintenance of the long axons. Long axons are like a circuit; they connect different areas of the brain from one brain cell to another in different areas. To give you an example, long axons run from the brain to our fingertips, all of which are myelinated (a protective cover or layer known as myelin). If cholesterol is lowered too much (e.g. by a statin drug), it can very easily promote transient global amnesia (TGA). When the cell membranes have too little cholesterol, nerve transmission or messaging can be affected. If we block or inhibit the body's ability to produce its own cholesterol, this will, in turn, inhibit the ability of the body to make its own neurosteroids. Cholesterol is not a neutral or innocuous molecule and is certainly not something that should be eliminated. Research shows that with a higher cholesterol level, the lower the incidence of Alzheimer's. This could be because they have more precursors to produce their own neurosteroids. Cholesterol is a powerful antioxidant and is **neuroprotective.**

So much so that the liver synthesizes the bloody stuff (sorry about that but... well, come on!) along with triglycerides (commonly known as fats) so they can be transported all over the body! The cholesterol that is not needed is transported back to the liver where it is converted into bile salts, which is part of bile, so it can be eliminated in feces. Not all of the cholesterol that is put into bile is necessarily excreted out of the body, some of it will be reabsorbed and then processed and reused as needed. It seems that cholesterol is such a vital molecule that the body even has a committed transport system, enabling it to deliver cholesterol all around the body, as needed. Here we have a question mark, or two... or three? Why would the body reuse cholesterol if it were so bad for our health? Why would it have a committed transport system? Why have cholesterol in the body in the first place?

Bile – here's another question mark. Cholesterol is a key component of bile. The liver produces approximately 75% of the body's cholesterol and about 70% of this is used to make bile. Bile is also made up of hormones, bile salts and toxins. Bile is stored in the gallbladder between meals and is part of the digestive mechanism; the gallbladder is pear-shaped and is situated just below the liver.

Gallbladder (1); Liver (2)

When food enters the duodenum, a release signal is sent to the gallbladder to squirt bile into the small intestines to help with the digestion and distribution of all lipids, including cholesterol, taken in through diet – not just greasy foods but healthy essential fats such as omega-3 fatty acids. Without bile, this process could not take place. Nearly all the cholesterol that reaches the gut, about 97% of it, is absorbed straight back into the bloodstream and sent back to the liver for processing. Bile, of course, has other functions as well, such as aiding the absorption of fat-soluble vitamins and dividing up endotoxins to prevent entry into the bloodstream. Endotoxins are toxins, as the word suggests, or bacteria. They are a part of the cell wall of microorganisms (bacteria).

Cholesterol has an important link to the immune system and is an important weapon in fighting infections. Cholesterol helps to neutralize toxins that are produced by bacteria and may leak into the bloodstream from the intestines (gut) if the immune system is weak and not functioning correctly. When there is infection in the body, total serum levels of cholesterol increase, but HDL (high-density lipoprotein, the supposed 'good' cholesterol of which we will talk more later) decreases. That is because it (HDL) is off on its crusade to fight the battle. Toxins cause damage. If you remember, cholesterol is vital for the routine repair of tissues, which is why it is found at the site of arterial injuries. Research shows that the so-called 'bad' cholesterol, or LDL, is able to inactivate more than 90% of the most toxic and, therefore, worst bacterial products.

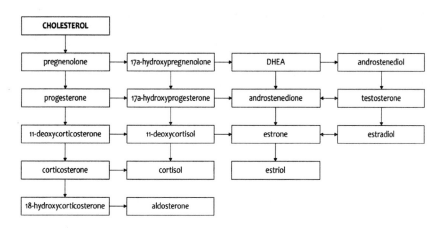

Biochemical Pathways of Steroid Hormones

So much so that it is the building block of all steroid hormones. Yes, a whole family of steroid hormones. These include cortisol and the entire tribe of sex hormones, including estrogens, progesterone and testosterone. These are known as the endogenous hormones – this simply means they are created by and in the body, which is a natural part of normal function, not to be confused with nasty synthetic hormones. No cholesterol, no hormones, no normal function… no party! If you want to party, you need cholesterol in the body. The first hormone to be manufactured is pregnenolone with the help of a specific enzyme (for every natural hormone there is an enzyme in between), which is the precursor to a cascade of other hormones, including the sex hormones.

How can we even begin to think we can be healthy without this vital substance in our body? Without cholesterol, the body will dysfunction and break down. To give you just one example of what can happen when cholesterol levels are very, very low, let's take a look at Smith-Lemli-Opitz Syndrome (SLOS). SLOS is a rare genetic syndrome where there is a defect in cholesterol synthesis, resulting in very low cholesterol levels. It is characterized by intellectual disability or learning problems, and behavioral problems; distinctive facial features and a small head size are also common. In children, it is common to see features of autism and malformations of lungs, heart, gastrointestinal tract, kidneys and genitalia. Infants experience feeding problems due to weak muscle tone (unable to suck well) and tend to grow and develop slower than other infants. The majority of affected individuals have fused second and third toes, and some may have extra fingers or toes. Hearing loss is common, cleft palate and eye abnormalities (cataracts and ptosis of eyelids) are also a feature.

How it works: mutations in the DHCR7 gene cause Smith-Lemli-Opitz Syndrome. The DHCR7 gene talks to or sends instructions for the enzyme 7-dehydrocholesterol reductase to be made. When mutations in this gene reduce or eliminate the activity of 7-dehydrocholesterol reductase, this prevents cells from producing enough cholesterol. The DHCR7 enzyme is responsible for the last step in the production of cholesterol. Cholesterol is necessary for correct embryonic development and has vital functions both before and after birth. And, with a lack of the DHCR7 enzyme, toxic byproducts of cholesterol production are allowed to accumulate in the blood, nervous system and other tissues. Last but not least, vitamin D3 is created from cholesterol. How, you might ask, is a vitamin made from cholesterol? Aren't vitamins usually procured from outside the body, from such things as food? Well, vitamin D3 is actually a hormone; it was wrongly named in times gone by. Let's take a quick look at how it is created. When sunlight hits the skin, 7-dehydrocholesterol is produced, which then converts into cholesterol, which in turn manufactures vitamin D3. Vitamin D3 plays a myriad of important roles in the body; the best known is its role in calcium metabolism and bone health. Importantly, it also protects against a number of cancers including breast, colon, skin and prostate. And, interestingly, compelling evidence links less than optimal vitamin D3 levels to heart disease. When vitamin D3 levels are optimal, its cardioprotective functions are invaluable, helping to keep inflammation away, normalize blood pressure and improve insulin sensitivity, all of which reduce cardiovascular disease risk.

So it would seem that cholesterol is a pretty important substance to have in the body, wouldn't it? Dot to dot! Cholesterol is there for a reason and not, by default, to give us a heart attack.

To recap: cholesterol helps make the coating of our cells, it protects our brain, makes up the bile salts (acids) that help to digest food in the intestines, it is important for the immune system, and it allows the body to make vitamin D and hormones such as pregnenolone, estrogens, testosterone and others. If cholesterol were not around, none of these functions would or could happen and, therefore, we humans would or could not exist. If cholesterol were not around, we could not produce the correct amounts of steroid hormones that enable us to stay healthy, both physically and mentally. In short, cholesterol is the building block of life.

It seems the dots are joining up and the question marks keep arriving. Something seems very wrong. Things appear to be a little more than 'illogical'! If the body needs so much cholesterol to keep it up and running (for normal functioning physiology) and cholesterol is present everywhere in the body, why then is the whole world trying to lower it? It's a 'misguided crusade', as Dr Dzugan likes to explain it, spurred on by the press, advertisements for foods low in cholesterol, and by those fancy posters you see strewn around your doctor's office clearly indicating where artery blockage can occur.

3. UNDERSTANDING CHOLESTEROL BEYOND ITS NUMBERS

It is not elevated levels of total cholesterol and LDL that predict whether or not you are going to have a heart attack unless, of course, they are extremely high. In fact, elevated cholesterol, over time, is a perfect marker indicating that the body is not functioning correctly as a whole. This malfunction should be corrected, not suppressed; the lowering of cholesterol is not necessary. CLDs do not resolve, they in fact worsen the situation, leading to deleterious side effects. Also, elevated LDL-cholesterol levels can be an indicator of a metabolic problem such as diabetes or an infection. Dr Dzugan and I believe that an elevated cholesterol level is an innocent bystander doing what the body is requesting it to do: deliver cholesterol to the tissues.

Cholesterol is not inherently bad; high levels don't necessarily mean you are on the pathway to coronary heart disease, just as low levels do not predict heart health. Unfortunately, though, this dreadful myth about cholesterol numbers is so ingrained in our minds and our 'hearts' that it has become a horrific international obsession. What the aging human truly needs is a balanced approach to reduce cardiovascular disease – an approach that safely normalizes cholesterol levels, an approach without any of the side effects statin drugs have to offer.

The majority of cholesterol inside the body is manufactured by the body, with a lesser amount coming from food. This sole fact should be an indication that cholesterol is an extremely important substance to have in the body. 85%-95% of cholesterol in our blood is 'endogenous' or manufactured by our own cells (mostly the liver). 5%-15% comes from the food we eat. Let's think about this for a second, please! In light of these percentages, could very low or zero cholesterol possibly then be good for the upkeep of our health? We think not; in fact, we know not! Low levels, or high levels for that matter, of cholesterol do not predict heart health.

As stated previously, cholesterol is a necessary building block of just about every system in the body and without it we would not survive. Cholesterol is a biological necessity, not a criminal. Having modest or even moderately elevated cholesterol levels doesn't necessarily mean that they will damage or cause harm to the arteries. And indeed, in many cases, when total cholesterol levels are high, it is the body's way of protecting itself from chronic infection and toxins. The logical side of your body is at work. Extra cholesterol floating in the bloodstream doesn't necessarily mean cardiovascular disease is on its way or is going to get worse.

To get a better understanding of how cholesterol works within the body, let's take a look at the body's committed transport system, which we spoke of earlier, and find out how it functions.

The Body's Committed Transport System of Cholesterol

We believe that most people are unaware of how intricate and delicate the body really is. Each system is tightly controlled by way of a feedback loop mechanism and has to work in harmony for us to be truly well. When there is an imbalance in any one of these systems, we will feel it; the body is continually talking to itself, trying to maintain homeostasis. Cholesterol is a molecule that is needed to keep these systems up and running and functioning perfectly. The human body's infrastructure rigidly controls cholesterol synthesis and absorption, along with its degradation. At this point, we pose this question: if cholesterol were such a bad molecule to have in the body, then why on earth would the body have a dedicated and highly intricate mechanism built into it? It wouldn't!

Cholesterol is oil-based; it is usually classified as a lipid and sometimes mistakenly referred to as a fat, which it is not. It is also known as a sterol, which is a combination of a steroid and an alcohol but, of course, it does not behave like alcohol. Cholesterol flows through the bloodstream (circulatory system) wrapped in packages made up of protein-covered particles appropriately named lipoproteins. The reason the body parcels cholesterol up into these packages is because cholesterol is oil-based and blood is water-based, so they don't mix well. Imagine dropping a few drops of olive oil into water. What happens? They float around and form globules, going nowhere or even somewhere they shouldn't.

These packages facilitate the transportation of lipoproteins in the blood, delivering them to the various workstations to be used when requested, or needed, by the body. Their actual job is to act as carriers for insoluble cholesterol and triglycerides (TRG).

Triglycerides are almost always grouped together as three fats, hence the 'tri' bit, meaning three, while 'glyceride' or glycerol is the backbone molecule that holds the fats together. Triglycerides are a type of fat found in the blood and are an all-important factor in the amount of energy they can generate. After a meal, the body converts excess calories into triglycerides. Triglycerides are deposited in the fat cells and are broken down for energy when the body requires them. In terms of energy storage, triglycerides produce more energy than carbohydrates and are also an important part of the chain of lipid carriers. Once they have completed their task, they can then be reabsorbed for storage or utilized as energy.

Similarly to LDL, triglycerides have also been seen to have anti-infective properties. Research shows that triglyceride-rich lipoproteins (VLDL and chylomicrons) can bind, neutralize and modulate the overall host response to bacterial endotoxins. In other words, in order to help fight infections, the body produces more triglycerides and LDLs. Interestingly, researchers have demonstrated that bacterial sepsis is linked to elevated triglycerides and other lipoprotein levels.

There are various types of lipoproteins, each in varying sizes, but the most well-known lipoproteins are HDL (high-density lipoprotein), which conventional medicine considers 'good' cholesterol, and LDL (low-density lipoprotein), which conventional medicine considers 'bad' cholesterol. The difference is in the ratio of protein to lipid. The more lipids to proteins the packages have, the lower the density, and the more proteins to lipids, the higher the density. Generally, lipoproteins are made up of proteins, phospholipids, cholesteryl ester, cholesterol and triglycerides.

To start off with, let's take a look at chylomicron, which is also a lipoprotein (although the name does not suggest that) and is the biggest of the bunch. Chylomicrons come from the Greek word *chylo* meaning 'milky' ('fluid-like') and *micron* meaning 'small size'. This lipoprotein transports lipids and cholesterol from the intestines, or gut, to the skeletal muscle and fat cells (adipose tissue) in the body. To give you a basic insight: after a meal, chylomicrons fill up with triglycerides, together with a small quantity of cholesterol; once they reach the fat cells, the triglyceride part is sucked away, leaving the chylomicron rather wizened. The shriveled chylomicron is then transported to the liver where it becomes a very-low-density lipoprotein (VLDL) and sent into the bloodstream. Chylomicrons consist of approximately 85%-88% triglycerides, 3% cholesteryl ester, 1% cholesterol, 8% phospholipids and 1%-2% proteins. They are the least dense of the transport particles as they carry a very small amount of protein.

VLDL (very-low-density lipoprotein) is another carrier which transports a high percentage of triglycerides (TRG) and a smaller percentage of the other components (hence the reason it is a very low lipoprotein – more fat-to-protein ratio). A key difference between VLDL and chylomicrons is that VLDL transports endogenous (made in the body) products, whereas chylomicrons transport exogenous (dietary) products. VLDL carries new synthesized triglycerides (TRG) from the liver to adipose tissue. As this carrier passes through the circulation, the triglyceride component is removed and is either stored as fat or used as fuel. Triglycerides are important 'players' in heart disease as high levels can increase the risk of cardiovascular problems but, again, please remember they also generate energy and have fighting powers against infections! A change of lifestyle and the addition of omega-3 fatty acids (fish oils), or preferably krill oils which contain phospholipid complex that increases absorption, can help lower triglyceride levels. Once VLDL has lost its triglyceride content, it becomes an intermediate-density-lipoprotein (IDL) particle. VLDL consists of approximately 50%-55% triglycerides, 12%-15% cholesteryl esters, 8%-10% cholesterol, 18%-20% phospholipids and 5%-12% protein. VLDL is smaller than chylomicrons but slightly denser.

IDL are short-lived and are composed of approximately 32%-35% cholesteryl esters, 8% cholesterol, 24%-30% triglycerides, 25%-27% phospholipids and 10%-12% protein. IDL are taken back into the liver for the purpose of reprocessing or losing more triglyceride content to become LDL. The size of IDL is smaller than VLDL and its density is between that of VLDL and LDL.

LDL is the primary plasma carrier and delivery service of cholesterol from the liver to the tissues or parts of the body that need it at any given time, where it is then absorbed by the cells all around the body. Along with being the primary carrier of cholesterol, it also accounts for transporting more than half of lipids circulating in the blood. LDL is also responsible for bringing cholesterol to production sites where it is needed (note the word 'needed'). LDL transports cholesterol which is both taken in via foods (exogenous) and produced within the body (endogenous). LDL consists of approximately 37%-48% cholesteryl esters, 8%-10% cholesterol, 10%-15% triglycerides, 20%-28% phospholipids and 20%-22% protein. And, of course, to be expected, it is smaller than IDL.

HDL is made in the intestines and the liver and acts like a sponge or vacuum cleaner which sucks up excess cholesterol that is not used by the tissues or cells, taking it back to the liver (this pathway is sometimes referred to as 'reverse cholesterol transport') where the HDL particle is reassembled, following which the cholesterol is either recycled or excreted into the bile. HDL consists of approximately 15%-30% cholesteryl esters, 2%-10% cholesterol, 3%-15% triglycerides, 24%-46% phospholipids and 55% protein.

All the varying types of lipoproteins transport the aforementioned components (proteins, phospholipids, cholesteryl ester, cholesterol and triglycerides) but carry different percentages of each component. It should be noted, though, that the percentages written above are only guidelines rather than fixed percentages. Guidelines, because these percentages are dependent on the body's requirements: each carrier has a specific job and the components that it carries are dependent on what is required or needs to be transported, where, and at a specific time. They are constantly in flux. It does not necessarily mean that the lipoproteins are always working at full capacity, rather, they are regulated by the body's requirements. The body is an incredible machine that is always looking out for itself and working to achieve homeostasis.

So, as you will have understood, the two major 'players' in the cholesterol story, LDL (the supposedly 'bad' cholesterol) and HDL (the supposedly 'good' cholesterol), are not actually cholesterol but transporters of cholesterol and other components. They have been wrongly named – they are carriers and are doing a job where one assists the other in an attempt to maintain balance. It is quite clear that both these carriers have different tasks and play different roles in the body – they have no conception of good or bad. They are working to maintain harmony and functionality within the body and have a very important physiological function. When the cells are in need of cholesterol, a signal is sent to the LDLs to deliver more cholesterol. Remember, they carry cholesterol from the liver, where it is made, to the tissues of the body. HDLs, on the other hand, are responsible for retrieving excess cholesterol in the periphery and taking it back to the liver. They are doing a job!

Lipoproteins carry various components and do not always work at full capacity, so the arbitrary figures of 50% (LDL) and 30% (HDL) of cholesterol in these two carriers are insignificant. It is therefore impossible to measure cholesterol directly in the bloodstream. The standard cholesterol panel only gives you a calculated measurement. "We don't know about you, but we find this terrifying." The medical industry is measuring cholesterol levels that cannot realistically be measured, and then it is blithely handing out statin drugs that are not required, whichever way you look at it.

The Standard Cholesterol Panel

It is worth taking a look at how conventional medicine measures cholesterol levels so you can better understand where they are coming from. Total cholesterol numbers are the numbers that supposedly have to be brought down to lessen your risk of a heart attack. As LDL carries the majority of cholesterol to the cells of the body, when blood tests are done, the amount of total cholesterol will reflect LDL levels, meaning a higher total cholesterol will reflect higher LDL levels. Likewise, when there is a lower total cholesterol level, there will be a lower LDL level. But let's take a closer look at these measurements.

$$LDL + HDL + (Triglycerides/5) = Total Cholesterol$$

At a glance, the word 'triglycerides' jumps off the page. What on earth have triglycerides got to do with cholesterol measurements? Are they one and the same? No, definitely not; triglycerides are triglycerides. But, like we said, cholesterol levels are a calculated measure, not a precise one. The division of triglycerides by five is the way in which VLDL is estimated. It assumes that virtually all of the plasma TG is carried on VLDL and that the cholesterol ratio is constant (about 5:1), which is not strictly so. So, in essence, the formula is:

$$LDL + HDL + VLDL = Total\ Cholesterol$$

However, VLDL is not always tested, even though, in order to obtain a 'total-cholesterol' value, the triglycerides are always divided by five. Confusing? No. It's just an estimate, not a true figure. There is another point of confusion in the above equation: nowhere is there any mention of cholesterol, just the LDL, HDL and VLDL carriers.

There is also another equation that comes into play here, the so-called 'Friedewald equation', which is used to calculate LDL (the supposedly 'bad' cholesterol):

$$Total\ Cholesterol - (Triglycerides/5 + HDL) = LDL$$

Of course, this equation has limitations as well. If the triglyceride level is higher than 400 mg/dL, then LDL cannot be measured accurately because concentrations higher than 400 mg/dL make the laboratory samples too thick. Another thing: if chylomicrons are present in the sample, they can interfere with accurate readings as well. Even when the equation is measured under optimal conditions, the amount of LDL can be miscalculated, being either underestimated or overestimated. This happens because the other tests are measured inaccurately as well, which obviously then goes on to create an imprecise measurement of LDL. Frightening! It all seems a bit lackadaisical to us, especially considering the damage CLD can do to the human body. In any event, whether we are trying to find LDL, HDL, VLDL or total cholesterol levels, we are not finding them because we are actually finding the estimates of the so-called carriers, which are carrying variable cholesterol levels.

Already, conventional medicine has spent huge amounts of money and time on failed research and is eternally debating which cholesterol is good and which is bad. There is no good or bad; cholesterol is an essential molecule and has a job to do. Apparently conventional medicine is now focusing its efforts on a test called VAP or LLP, which supposedly gives a more accurate measurement of lipoproteins. This test also measures the subtypes of lipoproteins (e.g. LDL, HDL and VLDL), such as HDL-3, HDL-2, VLDL-1, VLDL-2 and VLDL-3, and examines particle size. Restorative medicine believes that this test is a waste of time and money. The real debate should be: "Hold up, guys, we've got it all wrong. Don't you think we should be spending all this time and money on what really does cause heart disease? And, at this point, shouldn't we also be asking ourselves what really does provoke cholesterol levels to rise?" To answer that question for them, a hormonal imbalance for one! As well as infections and toxins, metabolic disorders such as diabetes and obesity. Why? Because the body is asking for more cholesterol production to help it out of a bad situation. The worst thing a doctor could do, at this point, is to offer a drug that blocks cholesterol production; which does not address the underlying cause.

Lipid subtypes, especially the number or concentration of small dense LDL particles, have been linked to the development of coronary-heart-disease events, but the data analysis of such studies is not adequate to show added benefits over risk assessment. Neither high LDL nor small LDL particle size causes heart disease – they are simply a warning sign that something is wrong (a dysfunction) in the body.

Evidence based on data obtained from multiple randomized clinical trials involving large numbers of patients showed that the measurement of lipid subtypes is not useful (and in some cases might be harmful). There is insufficient data that the measurement of lipid subtypes, over time, is useful to evaluate the effects of treatment.

We say it again: frightening! How is it possible that they can 'push' this cholesterol-lowering industry when they know the numbers obtained are not realistic and they are aware of the damage these CLDs cause? This is not very reassuring.

A Further Discussion of Subtypes

Subtypes of LDL, HDL and VLDL, of which there are many, examine particle size. Particle size is usually divided into two specific types, described as the small and dense type, and the large and buoyant type. The larger one carries more cholesterol, whilst the smaller one carries less cholesterol but is apparently more dangerous as the oxidized cholesterol can more easily slip through the endothelium and burrow into the artery walls, provoking the toxic brew even further. But what we need to remember here is that, again, if there is no 'scratch' (no damage), cholesterol, oxidized or not, will not attach to the endothelium. So the 'start point' of the problem (atherosclerosis) is not actually cholesterol but damage to the arterial structure.

Whatever, the key point to remember here is that cholesterol per se, oxidized or not, is not a demon; it is not something to be afraid of. Cholesterol and heart disease do not necessarily go hand in hand. Cholesterol that travels freely through the bloodstream is not a risk factor for the heart and its health, just as long as it stays in the bloodstream and does not rise to extremely high numbers. Gone are the days when we believed that, when total cholesterol numbers rose beyond a certain level, they 'got shoved' into the walls of the arteries just because the body didn't know what to do with it or where else to put it. We now know that, without that initial scratch, without that damage inside the artery walls, the human being can tolerate a fair amount of cholesterol in the bloodstream.

Understanding Oxidation

The word oxidation seems to suggest it must have something to do with oxygen. Well, kind of. The body needs oxygen; our cells need oxygen to produce energy. Without oxygen we would die; but the eternal and endless interaction with oxygen also stresses our body. This is the beginning of oxidation. Oxidation is a natural biochemical process which is continual and results in the production of free radicals – unbalanced molecules that interact with other molecules within the cells, which go on to damage cell membranes, proteins and genes. Free radicals cause the body's organs and systems to dysfunction and lose capacity. When they damage cell membranes, this affects the ability of the cells to transmit and receive messages from other cells, allowing the absorption of necessary nutrients and the elimination of waste products, for example. As we age, free radicals cause minimal but continuous deterioration of cells, organs and systems, eventually culminating in disease. The major danger is the havoc they can wreak when they react with important cellular components such as DNA and brain function, for example. This is called free-radical damage.

When the effect becomes excessive and uncontrolled, free-radical-induced oxidative stress occurs, which promotes the development of, and can worsen, many conditions, including heart disease, macular degeneration, diabetes and all cancers. Also, it is a well-known fact that oxidative stress or damage is a key factor of accelerated aging.

Just as inflammation is a necessary biochemical reaction to life, so is oxidation. It is only when the two get out of hand that problems can occur. When oxidation happens too often or the wrong substances become oxidized, we are moving one step closer to breakdown and chronic disease.

4. THE MYTH OF THE CHOLESTEROL DIET

Most, if not all, doctors, including cardiologists, believe that cholesterol, at any level, can cause heart disease – like we said: simple word, complex situation. Of course, we now know that this is not true. To better understand where this misleading hypothesis came from, we need to start at the beginning.

In 1926, Dr James B Herrick published the first US medical description of a heart attack. It was, at the time, a medical rarity and not something that made the medical community sit up and listen. In truth, it was not until after WWII that the medical community started to pay attention to heart disease when, suddenly, middle-aged men started falling backwards and not getting up again, in apparently epidemic proportions. In 1948, the World Health Organization (WHO) created the International Classification of Diseases (ICD) and, as a result, coronary heart disease (CHD) was born. Up until that point, different countries had different ways of classifying disease, so there were and are actually no true figures for a disease such as CHD before 1948. In fact, the French did not start using the ICD until 1968, twenty years later, so the term 'myocardial infarction' didn't exist in their language. Thus, by all accounts, CHD suddenly seemed to come about, and in plenty, after 1948; before that, people didn't die from it. The French were luckier though; they didn't start dying from it until after 1968. Is that possible? We'll let you answer that. The point is, the statistics that are placed in front of us should be looked at with skepticism. The statistics we get are not always the statistics that they seem. Looking at it logically, CHD must have existed before 1948 (and before 1968 for the French)!

As an example, in England, from 1930 to 1955, the mortality from heart attacks increased sixfold (while the intake of animal fat was unchanged, before the 'crazy' hypothesis!). How can we possibly know this when heart disease was not classified until after 1948? Please also remember that World War II was going on at the time, ending in 1945, which would surely have affected and/or obscured some of these numbers.

The History of the Cholesterol/Heart-Disease Hypothesis

The cholesterol/heart-disease hypothesis preaches that, when you consume too much cholesterol via diet, it causes a build-up of cholesterol and plaque in the arteries, which leads to atherosclerosis or hardening of the arteries (there are two words to describe this: incredibly wrong!). This, in turn, will cause an acute obstruction of coronary blood flow, which will result in a heart attack.

So, where and when did all this turmoil about cholesterol and its connection to heart disease begin? Precisely, in Berlin, in the mid-19th century. Rudolf Virchow, a German doctor and famous pathologist, was the first to introduce the lipid hypothesis, suggesting that blood-lipid accumulation in arterial walls was the cause of atherosclerosis or thickened plaques. In 1858, Virchow showed that cholesterol did not actually initiate the process, rather, it was the end product of degeneration. The most obvious sign observed was damage to the tissue then, after the damage occurred, an accumulation of fat appeared, a 'fatty streak'. As the scar tissue formed, a high amount of cholesterol then appeared. Remember, one of cholesterol's many jobs is to act as an agent of repair.

Another fifty years passed before any more significant interest was taken in heart disease. Dr Nikolai Anitschkov, a Russian researcher, was the next in line and had the 'not-such-a-clever idea' of using rabbits to prove his hypothesis. He fed them cholesterol to see the results in relation to plaque build-up in the arteries. Why was this not such a clever idea? Because rabbits are herbivores (plant eaters, in other words) and, as such, do not consume animal cholesterol in their natural diet. Dr Anitschkov did not consider this fact. Rabbits cannot utilize cholesterol effectively. The end result was quite terrible, in fact: anything from completely yellowed eyes to loss of fur occurred, as well as atherosclerosis in rabbits that were fed huge quantities of cholesterol. This was an extremely nonsensical study – rabbits are rabbits and like green grass, humans are humans and are carnivores. Basically, we have a completely different infrastructure. This was not a good time for accurate scientific research but, when people are so determined to 'push' a cholesterol hypothesis forward, results like this can appear convincing, even good. Whatever, he was one of the pioneers of the devastating cholesterol hypothesis we see today.

In 1950, John Gofman hypothesized that blood cholesterol was the main cause of coronary heart disease (CHD) and then, a year later, Duff and McMillan created the lipid hypothesis in its modern form. A few years later, in 1953, a young Ancel Keys, spurred on by the lipid hypothesis, published a paper that discussed saturated fats and cholesterol as the cause of heart disease. Initially, he thought that dietary fat in general caused cholesterol levels to rise but, as the years passed, he then began to believe that it was specifically saturated fat that caused cholesterol levels to rise. Today, this brilliant idea (tongue in cheek) that saturated fat is the true criminal is so ingrained in our minds that even most health writers cannot write the words 'saturated fat' without adding the words 'artery-clogging'. So untrue! Put simply, this is the basis of the lipid hypothesis that has been thrown at us for more than fifty years: saturated fat drives up cholesterol levels; elevated cholesterol levels lead to heart disease. A very easy and very simple theory, but not true. This hypothesis, which, by the way, has never been proven, is a 'scientific swindle'!

Cholesterol Paranoia

Since Keys believed that fat in the diet and cholesterol in the blood were linked, he devised the 'Seven Countries Study' to prove his hypothesis. He took data from various countries and looked at fat consumption and its connection to heart disease. He then published the results of this famous study that supposedly showed a linear correlation between the amount of dietary-fat consumption and the incidence of cardiovascular disease. The results seemed pretty clear, the evidence was there, he had proved his point: fat consumption drives up cholesterol and elevated cholesterol causes heart disease. Where there is a will, there is always a way! But things weren't as simple as that. This study was, instead, as we like to call it, a 'non-scientific swindle hypothesis'. This study was completely and utterly a fraud! And, unfortunately, it was this study that 'set in stone' the recommendations of the low-fat-diet/heart-disease hypothesis we see today. It is therefore worth taking a quick but closer look at it, to see how things really went.

Although it was known as the 'Seven Countries Study', Keys actually had data from twenty-two countries at his disposal but, out of these, he cherry-picked seven and examined the consumption of saturated fat (fats that are solid at room temperature, mostly found in dairy products and meat). To his amazement (we are being sarcastic), he found a straight-line relationship between heart disease, cholesterol levels and saturated fat intake. The seven countries were: Italy, Greece, former Yugoslavia, Netherlands, Finland, USA and Japan. You will note we use the word 'cherry-picked' – that's because Keys explicitly chose those aforementioned countries so as to support his preconceived hypothesis. He could well have chosen another seven countries out of the twenty-two and proved the exact opposite. Keys desperately wanted to prove his point; therefore, he cherry-picked the data to prove that the more saturated fat people consumed, the higher the risk of heart disease. Had he chosen, for example, Finland, Israel, Netherlands, Germany, Switzerland, France and Sweden out of the twenty-two countries, the results would have been completely different – proving that there was no correlation to heart disease and dietary-fat consumption.

Although Keys' study was undoubtedly flawed, everyone, including the American Medical Association, the American Heart Association, nutritionists, and even the American Government, chose to believe his low-fat-diet/heart-disease hypothesis. Keys was a member of the nutrition advisory committee of the American Heart Association which, in 1961, embraced Ancel Keys' low-fat dietary recommendations. In 1980, the US Department of Agriculture released the very first 'Dietary Guidelines for Americans', stating that people should avoid too much fat, saturated fat and cholesterol. The low-fat diet became the 'sign of the times'. The whole Western world held hands and willingly joined the pandemonium. Cholesterol and healthy foods, such as butter and dairy products, were condemned to the depths of hell. These were the times when we all believed that fat, and in particular saturated fat, was the Devil himself because it would, in turn, clog the arteries, leading to a heart attack. (False!) These were the times when we were told that carbohydrates were needed for energy and for the survival of the fittest. (Totally untrue, of course!) We were told that saturated fats were dangerous.

In 1986-1987, the National Institute of Health announced a new program, called the National Cholesterol Education Program (NCEP), to fight the number-one killer, heart disease. Its goal was to reduce the prevalence of elevated cholesterol in the blood and, therefore, reduce coronary-heart-disease morbidity and mortality.

Study after Study, with No Evidence!

After 1961, a host of studies came flooding in: the Honolulu Heart Program and the Puerto Rico Heart Health Program are two examples. Neither of these studies showed any evidence that men on a low-fat diet lived any longer or had fewer heart attacks than men who ate a high-fat diet.

In 1970, one of the more important studies, the infamous Framingham Heart Study, conducted a study entitled 'Diet and the Regulation of Serum Cholesterol'. The researchers involved intended to prove that it was, indeed, the food consumed that caused high cholesterol levels. To measure this, they selected 912 men and women and compared the amount of cholesterol they consumed in their diet with the cholesterol levels in their blood. To their surprise, they found that there was no relationship. They then went on to study how much saturated fat and calories these individuals ate. Again, there was no relationship between cholesterol levels and diet.

Dr William Kannel and Dr Tavia Gordon, two of the researchers, then went on to report that "these findings suggest a cautionary note with respect to hypotheses relating diet to serum cholesterol levels", as they wrote in their summary. "There is a considerable range of serum cholesterol levels within the Framingham Study Group. Something explains this inter-individual variation, but it is not diet." The researchers concluded that: "There is, in short, no suggestion of any relation between diet and the subsequent development of CHD in the study group." Unfortunately, this study was never published! One should ask why but, of course, we know why.

There were many more studies that showed little to no relationship between the amount of cholesterol in the diet and the development of atherosclerosis and coronary heart disease. As an example, in 1991 two researchers reviewed sixteen trials to evaluate the impact that diet had on serum cholesterol. The results showed that lowering the amount of cholesterol one ate only reduced blood-cholesterol levels by no more than 4% when following the dietary recommendations set forth by the National Heart, Lung and Blood Association's National Cholesterol Education Program (NCEP) – the same recommendations endorsed by the American Heart Association. These guidelines were intended for people who had high cholesterol (hypercholesterolemia) and entailed a restriction of total fat intake per day to no more than 30% of total calories, saturated fat intake to no more than 10% of total calories and cholesterol to less than 300 mg/day. The only problem is/was (whether it is the year 2016 or was the year 1991, our body's infrastructure remains the same), these guidelines have and have had little impact on cholesterol levels. We should also take a look at the studies of different cultures in which people routinely consume high amounts of saturated fat and cholesterol, such as many of the African tribes. As an example, the Samburus consume more than twice the amount of animal fat than the average American or European but their cholesterol levels are only about 170 mg/dL. The Masai in Kenya consume large amounts of high-fat Zebu milk daily, yet their cholesterol levels are among the lowest recorded in the world. At this point it could be argued that low cholesterol is inherited among these cultures. A study of Masai tribesmen who moved to the city of Nairobi, where they consumed a much lower cholesterol diet, showed that their new diet did not lower their cholesterol any further.

Simply put, diet does not cause high cholesterol, nor does it have a significant impact on cholesterol levels. To understand better, let's take a look at the 'cholesterol feedback mechanism' and see how it functions to strictly control cholesterol regulation.

The Cholesterol Feedback Mechanism

(To have knowledge is to understand; to understand is to have power.)

Why does the cholesterol we eat have a minimal effect on serum cholesterol? Because the body regulates cholesterol levels in the liver according to each individual's requirements. The more cholesterol one eats, the less the liver makes, and vice versa.

The human liver synthesizes roughly 3,000 mg of new cholesterol in a twenty-four-hour period and the majority of people can handle an intake of cholesterol within the range that people usually consume, namely 300 mg to 400 mg, without any significant alteration in blood-cholesterol levels. People usually get 5%-15% of cholesterol through their diet; however, in most people, less than 5% of cholesterol in the bloodstream gets there through diet. As stated previously, the human body's infrastructure rigidly controls cholesterol synthesis and absorption, along with its degradation. The body is set up in a way to naturally protect us, not naturally harm us. Why is it then that we are consistently being told to reduce cholesterol levels?

At this point, considering the aforementioned calculations, going all out and searching for foods low in cholesterol would seem to be pretty ridiculous. And trying to lower cholesterol by way of diet would seem absurd and, in fact, a waste of time. If we decrease our consumption of cholesterol through food, the actual effect on blood is minute because, when we cut down on cholesterol, the body naturally increases its production to make up for the missing source. In other words, if we eat less cholesterol, the liver produces more, and if we eat more cholesterol, the liver produces less – simple as that. Cholesterol is primarily made in the liver, which is the 'central production plant', and it is the liver that is responsible for the seesaw setup of 'consume more/make less' or 'consume less/make more'. There is a 'feedback point'; the body is always trying to balance itself to maintain homeostasis.

The Criminal Content of a Vote

The cholesterol/heart-disease story is truly a mix of personalities, from the well-meaning but misguided to the gangsters and fraudsters that keep the cholesterol myth up and running today. It is an all-powerful and well-cultivated myth with some very determined industries behind it, industries that make billions of dollars at a time – the statin and food industries, for two!

In 1973, the NIH initiated and funded a trial called the Lipid Research Clinic's Coronary Primary Prevention Trial (LRC-CPPT). Primary prevention is classed as an attempt to prevent heart disease or heart attack ever occurring, whereas secondary prevention is when a person already has heart disease or has suffered a heart attack. It is important to understand the difference between primary and secondary prevention, as we will mention it throughout the book. The goal of this primary prevention trial was to lower cholesterol levels with the use of a cholesterol-lowering drug (cholestyramine which, at full dosage (24 g/day), reduced total blood cholesterol by 20%-25% and

LDL cholesterol by 30%-35%) rather than through diet. In *their* minds, lowering cholesterol by diet or by a drug was the same thing just as long as *they* lowered cholesterol levels. Naturally, this medicine did lower cholesterol, that was its purpose, i.e. to inhibit cholesterol production, and it did modestly reduce heart-disease rates in the process and the probability of dying from a heart attack over a seven-year period, although there was no decrease in total mortality rates. This outcome is what true researchers call a 'statistical significance', which translates into 'chance'. It is barely enough and is not hard evidence. Nevertheless, it was enough to push the lipid hypothesis one step further (or backward, as the case may be), lowering cholesterol by way of a drug. Whatever, in their opinion, it proved cholesterol had to be lowered to escape heart disease.

In 1984, the NIH held a 'consensus-development conference' to clarify and try to stipulate the results of the LRC-CPPT along with dietary recommendations. One would hope, pray, presume and assume that we lived in a world that was fair and just, in a world where new and dynamic scientific data was accepted only after rigorous testing had been done, and where overwhelming evidence was delivered. Not so! This supposed scientific consensus was far from being scientific. Usually, in these types of consensus, specific scientific questions are listed and then addressed. In this case, the list of questions addressed was:

- Is the relationship between blood-cholesterol levels and coronary heart disease causal?
- Will reduction of blood-cholesterol levels help prevent coronary heart disease?
- Under what circumstances and at what level of blood cholesterol should dietary or drug treatment be started?
- Should an attempt be made to reduce the blood-cholesterol levels of the general population?
- What research directions should be pursued on the relationship between blood cholesterol and coronary heart disease?
- These are not scientific questions. The real question is: should a consensus be based on a survey of results or on a specific scientific method?
- It is important to note that several experts questioned various issues of the trials and even questioned their accuracy. However, the final report made it seem like everyone had agreed on the 'cholesterol-

must-be-lowered-to-avoid-heart-disease' concept, either by diet or by a drug. They were good to go!

Note: In 1978, six years before the consensus-development conference, Dr Kaare R Norum of the University of Oslo conducted a survey to define whether there was a consensus among experts on atherosclerosis, its relation to blood-cholesterol levels and the development of heart disease; and whether or not the knowledge available surrounding diet and heart disease was sufficient to recommend a change in diet. A questionnaire was sent to 211 prominent researchers, including epidemiologists, nutritionists, geneticists and many others who were researching lipids and atherosclerosis at that time. 90% answered with the affirmative and the other 10% were either not sure or they did not agree. Again, a general question such as this cannot be classed as a scientific question, therefore, cannot be answered in a scientific way. Science is based on accuracy of observations and statements made. It is a complex chain of rigorous testing involving numerous parties which reinforce this accuracy. A survey does not replace the observation and accuracy of science. To find the truth, you cannot be a voter – one needs to be an observer, an investigator and an analyst in order to be able to reach a conclusive hypothesis.

Armed and Extremely Dangerous!

In 1987, armed with the so-called results of the CPPT and the supposedly unified consensus, the National Heart, Lung and Blood Institute (NHLBI) announced the setting up of the National Cholesterol Education Program (NCEP) to help fight the number-one killer, heart disease, advising the public that, if they wanted to be healthy and heart-disease-free, they should reduce elevated cholesterol levels in the blood, which would reduce coronary-heart-disease morbidity and mortality. The show must go on! Literally and suddenly, millions of people were catapulted into another world believing they were, and had been, walking around with a severe medical condition – high cholesterol – that needed treatment. They were told that the cause of heart disease had been found and a true treatment was now available – if diet wouldn't cure it, a drug would. Cholesterol-lowering drugs were introduced in the 1980s but became more largely available in the mid-1990s.

The fact that the NHLBI decided to launch this program on its own authority and specifically hand-picked the panel's specialists speaks volumes. There was no White House approval, nor was it passed by Congress for review! Again, we repeat ourselves, one would have thought that, before introducing such a program to millions of people and moving forward with such a medication, sound scientific testing would have been done to ensure it was safe and effective. No such testing was done.

The Ever-Declining Levels of Cholesterol

The recommended levels of cholesterol have been declining consistently over the years; but what is meant by recommended cholesterol levels? Who decides, what is the recommended level and what is not the recommended level? As we asked in chapter 2, is a level not a level? Do we humans change so dramatically and continually, do our cholesterol levels fluctuate so drastically year in, year out that the pharmaceutical industries are obliged to adjust these levels accordingly or to an ever-decreasing baseline? If, for thousands of years, the human biochemistry has been reasonably stable, should we not then be researching and studying the 'whys', 'whats' and 'hows' that support and reinforce the human biochemical pathways, instead of trying to disrupt them with such drugs as statins? The mechanism of most drugs is to either inhibit crucial enzymes or to block receptors, neither of which is natural and will cause a chain reaction of confusion within the body.

Currently, according to the conventional guidelines set by the National Heart, Lung and Blood Institute, recommended levels are as follows: 240 mg/dL or greater is considered high cholesterol, with 200 mg/dL or lower being 'ideal' and everything in between considered 'borderline high'. Where are these levels coming from? Certainly not through rigorous scientific testing but, more likely, through 'a rigorous voting system' and financial gain.

A normal reference range for a particular test or measurement is usually defined as the value that 95% of the population falls into. The whole point of a normal range is to describe the majority of people or the 'normal' part of the population (95%), while taking into account the fringe members (5%) who do not fall under this range. So, if we say that hypercholesterolemia is 300 mg/dL and above, but decide to move that number down by 100 mg/dL, we have just corrupted the concept of normal ranges. This 'corrupted' normal range can no longer be considered a normal range but a recommended range. Suddenly, with an extra buffer of 100 mg/dL, a significantly larger percentage of the population 'qualifies' for a cholesterol-lowering drug, which will greatly increase financial gain for those involved in the statin industry.

Prior to 1980, the normal range for hypercholesterolemia was defined as 210 mg/dL in individuals younger than twenty years of age to more than 280 mg/dL in individuals older than sixty years of age. In 1970, the normal range for cholesterol was 150-280 mg/dL. In 1990, the desirable blood-cholesterol value became anything below 200 mg/dL. In 1995, the normal range of cholesterol became 150-250 mg/dL. In 1996, the recommended range became anything below 200 mg/dL. In 2002, the focus was on LDL and any range below 100 mg/dL was considered optimal. However, 5% (fringe members) of the population in Western countries have a total cholesterol higher than 300 mg/dL. According to the definition of normal ranges, this should be classed as true hypercholesterolemia (this figure is roughly 20% lower among Asians) but, according to the recommendations presented by the medical industries, this value should be 200 mg/dL or below. Here we have to ask yet again: why? Perhaps it is the 'extra-buffer' situation again!

In 2004, when the National Cholesterol Education Program lowered recommended cholesterol levels (yet again), eight out of the nine people on the panel had financial ties to the pharmaceutical industries, most of them being manufacturers of cholesterol-lowering drugs who would immediately reap benefits from these new recommendations. Up until then, recommended LDL levels of less than 130 mg/dL were considered low enough but these new guidelines called for extra cholesterol monitoring and treatment which, in fact, recommended that LDL should be 70 mg/dL in patients at high risk for heart disease. It is actually almost impossible for most individuals to have LDL levels of 70 mg/dL unless they are very sick or dying of cancer, or unless they are on aggressive cholesterol-lowering medication. Patients quite frequently have to take more than one cholesterol-lowering drug to achieve these targets. Sound ominous? People whose cholesterol levels drop below

45 mg/dL would simply not survive. Severe hypocholesterolemia may serve as a clinically useful prognostic parameter. At this point it is not a question of a few side effects here and there or catching a cold or the flu – they would simply expire.

An interesting point to make here is that the majority of studies use the terms 'LDL Cholesterol' and 'HDL Cholesterol' even though these carriers are NOT cholesterol. If you recall from earlier on in this chapter, we mentioned that lipoproteins consist of a mix of proteins, phospholipids, cholesteryl ester, cholesterol and triglycerides. Confusing? Not really. It is done with purpose behind it!

In 2011, the American National Heart, Lung and Blood Institute (NHLBI) issued new guidelines introducing statin use to reduce heart disease in young adults and teenagers if cholesterol was at a certain level. According to a recent study done in April 2015, this would mean that nearly half a million teens and young adults, between the ages of seventeen and twenty-one, would qualify for statin treatment. Incredible! We should take a step back for a second and examine this logically, as all is not as it seems. As stated previously, cholesterol (we like to think of this as the manufacturing plant) produces a cascade of steroid hormones. Hormones are the single most powerful messaging machine in the human body and are part of what keeps us up and running and the body functioning correctly (we will discuss hormones in depth and how important they are to physiological function in the following chapters). What are our children going to do without hormones? How can they possibly function and stay healthy when hormone production is interrupted?

In various studies, hypercholesterolemia was found in up to 53.1% of schoolchildren. At this point we should question: are children dropping like flies because of atherosclerosis? No. So there must be something else, something more logical, involved in elevated cholesterol levels – and, of course, there is! These levels are simply a natural response and progression of human development, which is also seen in pregnancies. For the regular growth of children and their development into adulthood, an extra amount of anabolic hormones is needed. When extra hormones are needed, at any time, the body will instinctively increase cholesterol production in order to secrete more hormones – it is a feedback mechanism. In pregnancies, total cholesterol and LDL levels increase significantly, along with triglycerides, because it is vital for the growth of the fetus. Following delivery, total cholesterol decreases significantly within three months and a further decrease occurs during the following nine months. There is also an increase in the amount of steroid hormones in the female body during pregnancy because she requires hormones, both for herself and for the growth of the child. This is what is called a biological response. If the body is unable to increase cholesterol and there are diminished concentrations of total cholesterol and LDL, a miscarriage may result. We repeat ourselves: what are our children going to do without cholesterol and, therefore, hormones?

2013: A New Set of Guidelines!

(The American College of Cardiology and American Heart Association Treatment of Blood Cholesterol to Reduce Atherosclerotic Cardiovascular Risk in Adults)

After the release of the ever-changing guidelines in 2013, things were looking good for the statin industries only! The only and best way to prevent heart disease, according to them, was to follow these new guidelines. These guidelines stated that the new cardiovascular prevention measures were decided upon only after years of scientific research which helped them in developing the most beneficial approaches to preventing heart disease and stroke. Some research! Remember, heart disease is the leading cause of death in the world. If statins are supposedly solving the heart-disease problem, why is it, then, that it is still the number-one killer? As already stated, statins were introduced in the 1980s but became widely prescribed in the 1990s; by 2005, millions of people were taking them. This fact alone should make you ask: "What the hell is going on?" If statins work, why haven't they reduced the incidence of heart-attack mortality?

Statins do not work; they have a 99% failure rate of reducing mortality! Statin defenders use the relative risk ratio to amplify the use of statins. If we were to look at the absolute risk, we would see that statin drugs benefit just 1% of the population, meaning that, out of one hundred people, one single individual will have one less heart attack. Not looking so good, especially if we consider the deleterious side effects that come with the statin drugs (we will discuss side effects in the following chapters). But, by making statistical maneuvers such as using the relative risk ratio, statins could be seen to be beneficial for 30%-50% of the population. The most important number a doctor can have in front of him/her is the absolute risk ratio, and, in fact, the relative risk ratio is completely senseless without absolute risk ratios.

To give you an example of how statistics can be manipulated to acquire the recommended levels, the JUPITER trial (Justification for the Use of Statins in Primary Prevention), which began in 2003 but ended early for unexplained reasons, declared to the public and healthcare workers that there was a 54% reduction in heart attacks. However, the authors of a study that examined the transparency and the deception of JUPITER noted: "The public and healthcare workers were informed of a 54 percent reduction in heart attacks, when the actual effect in reduction of coronary events was less than 1 percentage point." How convenient!

Two years after the original study was released, the Archives of Internal Medicine published three studies (one of which is mentioned above) discrediting the claims that had been defined by the industry-sponsored JUPITER study. JUPITER was funded by Astra-Zeneca, which is the maker of Crestor (a statin drug) – nine out of fourteen authors had financial ties to Astra-Zeneca. Of course, at this point, one couldn't expect anything other than a beneficial outcome for the statin industries. At long last, the JUPITER trial was being scrutinized, as it should have been from its initiation, especially because of how instrumental it was to revving up sales of statins. Initially, statins were to be prescribed for secondary prevention, but the JUPITER trial opened up a whole new market by claiming statins could be of "significant benefit" when used for primary prevention as well.

Another of these studies discussed the method and results of this trial and proclaimed it as "flawed", stating that "the results do not support the use of statin treatment for primary prevention against cardiovascular disease".

Jumping Back to the New 2013 Guidelines

These new guidelines recommended that statins should be prescribed in four basic groups and seemed to require a simple 'yes' or 'no' as an answer! Let's take a look at these questions:

- Have you been diagnosed with clinical atherosclerotic coronary vascular disease?
- Is your LDL higher than 190 mg/dL?
- Do you have diabetes (type 1 or type 2) with LDL between 70-189 mg/dL?
- Is your ten-year risk factor of developing cardiac disease greater than 7.5%?

For the first time, the 2013 guidelines recommended statin use in primary prevention treatment as well as in secondary prevention. These new guidelines, again, opened up a whole new section for the statin industries and greatly increased the number of individuals who 'qualified' for a statin drug. Great profit margins! Also, please note that these guidelines did away with the previous recommendations of using the lowest dose of drug possible – this would typically mean you would be prescribed a low-dose statin drug together with one, or even two, more cholesterol-lowering drugs. Very convenient!

To get a better understanding of these recommended guidelines, let's take a quick look at each group.

Adults with Clinical Atherosclerotic Coronary Vascular Disease

As this group encompasses individuals who have already had a cardiovascular event, it focuses on secondary prevention (to prevent another cardiac event occurring). Let us just say again that statins have a very high failure rate – they do not work. They cannot save you from a second heart attack – or a first, come to that! Adults do not acquire atherosclerosis because they have a deficiency of a statin drug; they get it as time goes on because of age, a hormonal imbalance, a breakdown in physiology, heavy metal toxicity, poor diet, smoking, because of cumulative and consistent damage over time. As we previously stated in chapter 1, atherosclerosis is a physiological adaptation to vascular damage or injury and is part of a failed healing process. First comes the damage or injury to the tissue, then comes an accumulation of various powerful healing materials such as cholesterol. If we inhibit cholesterol by way of a statin drug, it cannot do its job – it can no longer protect us, heal our hearts, our body or our minds.

LDL Higher than 190 mg/dL

LDL is not the dangerous molecule that we've been led to believe it is. In fact, as we previously stated, it is an essential substance for every cell in the body. It helps fight infections and is an anti-inflammatory agent – in other words, it helps protect against damage. So why should we want to lower it to the recommended ranges? LDL is not the problem; it is just doing what the body is asking it to do, shuttling cholesterol from the liver to the tissues, fighting infection, acting as an anti-inflammatory molecule and protecting the arteries from the effects of cumulative damage.

Adults with Diabetes (Type 1 or Type 2) with LDL between 70-189 mg/dL

It is quite incredible that so many adults with diabetes are being recommended statins. Why? Because statins have been seen to increase the risk of developing type 2 diabetes. There are a great many studies indicating that statins increase diabetes and the longer you take them, the higher the risk. The JUPITER trial was one such study and showed that there was a 25% increased risk of new-onset diabetes in the group that took statins. Statins may actually lower cholesterol levels, which really are neither here nor there in the heart-disease connection, but they also increase blood-glucose levels (hyperglycemia) – it is a side effect of the statin medication. Statins affect, or rather, impair pancreatic-beta-cell function (where insulin is produced) and decrease insulin sensitivity; continual insulin sensitivity will eventually provoke type 2 diabetes (see chapter 1). Insulin is a hormone that reduces blood glucose (sugar). We need a certain amount of insulin to maintain balanced blood-glucose levels but too much of it is bad – elevated levels cause inflammation, which in turn causes damage. Statin drugs increase insulin levels, which is devastating not only to our health but to our heart; elevated insulin levels lead to heart disease. Let's think this one through. Isn't this why cholesterol-lowering drugs are prescribed in the first place…to protect against heart disease and heart attacks?

Another study published in the *Lancet*, which was named 'Statins and risk of incident diabetes: a collaborative meta-analysis of randomized statin trials' and began in 1994 and ended in 2009, showed that individuals treated with statins had a 9% increase for diabetes. 91,140 participants took either a statin or a placebo. However, this study did not take into account other factors such as pre-diabetes, so the 9% could actually have been higher than stated.

Ten-Year Risk Factor of Developing Cardiac Disease Greater than 7.5 Percent

Our first questions are: what is a 7.5% risk factor and who determines this restraint? Let's take a guess!

The ten-year heart-attack risk involves the use of an online calculator – yes, a calculator! An online cardiovascular calculator! Seems we do not need a doctor anymore. The recommendations state that, if your risk of developing cardiac disease is greater than 7.5% over a period of ten years, then you need a statin drug. By pulling out your computer and clicking onto the cardiovascular calculator, then pumping in your cholesterol and HDL numbers, your age and whether you smoke or not, you can find out if you need to take medication. Only problem is, this calculator has been seen to greatly overestimate the outcome by over 75%. It has purposely been 'fixed' to overestimate the results so as to ensure that millions more will be candidates for the statin drug. This setup is flawed, and it turns out that the majority of people, when using this calculator, have a greater than 7.5% risk.

When questioned why the cardiovascular calculator overestimated the results, the American Heart Association and the American College of Cardiology (the two organizations that published the guidelines) went on to say that, while the calculator was not perfect, it was a major step forward and that the guidelines already state that patients and doctors should discuss treatment options rather than blindly follow a calculator. We say: what is the point of a calculator in the first place if not to acquire more candidates for a statin drug? It certainly seems that way anyway.

As previously stated, statin drugs are not your way out of a heart attack or stroke, do not resolve the problem of heart disease and they certainly should not be used as a form of preventive medicine. They are dangerous and have numerous deleterious side effects, which we will discuss further in the following chapters.

A New Class of Drug: LDL 'Cholesterol'-Lowering Drugs

In July 2015, proprotein-convertase-subtilisin/kexin-type 9 (PCSK9) inhibitors were introduced both to lower LDL levels in individuals with familial hypercholesterolemia (an inherited condition which causes extremely high LDL levels – we will discuss this further in the following chapters) and for secondary prevention (patients who have already suffered a heart attack or stroke). On July 24th, 2015, the European Commission (EC) granted "permission to launch" this new class of drug onto the marketplace. Two days later, the Food and Drug Administration (FDA) followed suit. PCSK9 inhibitors are an injectable drug that works by increasing the liver's ability to bind and remove low-density lipoproteins (LDLs) from the blood. They disarm the function of PCSK9s which suppress the liver's reuptake of LDLs.

PCSK9 is an enzyme that causes degradation to the LDL receptor that binds to LDL and is basically a mechanism which keeps things in balance. LDL is extracted from the blood and absorbed into the cell; the LDL receptor then disintegrates, leaving everything in balance; if there is no LDL receptor, the LDL cholesterol then stays in the blood. PCSK9 inhibitors work by blocking the PCSK9 enzyme, which will then leave you with more LDL receptors on the cell surface (liver cells, in this case), which will allow for more LDL to be taken into the cell. This then leaves less cholesterol circulating in the bloodstream, which appears to be a good solution for the lowering of cholesterol, but the outcome is that the cells are then left overflowing with cholesterol, which is not a natural event. What are our cells going to do with all the cholesterol? This interferes with cell function, which will more than likely contribute to all types of dysfunction in the body. As stated previously, cholesterol is found in all cells of the body and all cells need cholesterol in their membranes – without it, they would/could not survive. It is the high amount of cholesterol found in these cell membranes that helps maintain their integrity and also facilitates cellular communication but what happens when there is an overload, an imbalance? The PCSK9 inhibitors have an entirely different mechanism from statins but this still does not mean that PCSK9 inhibitors are safe or won't produce side effects.

PCSK9 inhibitors hover on a very thin wire and are poised to create havoc within the body. A seventy-eight-week-long study, published in the *New England Journal of Medicine* in April 2015, showed that PCSK9 inhibitors caused a higher incidence of many of the same side effects as statins (we will discuss statins and their side effects in the following chapters). And it is worth mentioning that the outcome on cardiovascular mortality and morbidity has not yet been established for these drugs. Larger and long-term studies are needed to determine their safety and efficiency.

However, PCSK9 drugs do lower LDL, there is no disputing that fact; they do the job they were designed to do, i.e. lower LDL. But we should question what the issue is here: a lab value or heart disease? These are two very different scenarios! In the OSLER and ODYSSEY studies, the new drugs (evolocumab [Repatha, Amgen] and alirocumab [Praluent, Sanofi/Regeneron]) showed a high level of negative neurocognitive effects. The follow-up was only eleven months in the OSLER study and seventy-eight weeks in the ODYSSEY study. This timeframe is far too short: heart-disease prevention is not a two-year endeavor!

But, amazingly enough, the pharmaceutical industries are using this newer class of cholesterol-inhibiting drug as a new selling point, stating that many individuals cannot tolerate statins due to side effects. Before the arrival of this new medication, they hid, minimized or totally ignored these issues. Absolutely incredible!

It is the wish of pharmaceutical industries to reduce cholesterol levels by as much as 75% with the use of PCSK9 inhibitors in combination with a statin drug. And, while they have convinced the medical profession, along with the public, that LDL is 'bad' and the lower you go, the better, researchers have not yet determined how low that 'low' really should be! But, as we have already stated, cholesterol is the most abundant molecule in the body and without it we cannot survive. Truth be known, though, both high and low levels of cholesterol are not good, as both cause disturbances in the body. What we want is normalized cholesterol levels.

Beware of New Drugs on the Way

ETC-1002 is a drug that is not yet on the marketplace but scientists are always researching and looking for new kinds of medicine to lower cholesterol levels. Beware! The mechanism of this drug works inside the liver to change how the body uses cholesterol and fats. Incredible!

Cholesterylester-transfer-protein (CETP) inhibitors (anacetrapib and evacetrapib) raise HDL and lower LDL. Studies have previously linked these drugs to an increased risk of heart attacks and death but, apparently, scientists are now trying to create a more promising version. Promising, how? Oh, they do keep trying, don't they? We say again: beware!

We should remember that when we take or ingest a CLD, quite often we decrease cholesterol way below the point that the majority of healthy individuals had at a young age. In other words, we are violating a biological law when we use these drugs. The body needs cholesterol like a flower needs sunlight and water to flourish and bloom. It doesn't matter how you lower cholesterol, whether it be with the use of a statin drug, a PCSK9 inhibitor, diet or exercise – if your cholesterol drops too low, you will suffer health issues and you certainly won't bloom; in fact, quite the opposite!

5. HIGH AND LOW CHOLESTEROL LEVELS AND RELATED PROBLEMS

We've already understood that conventional medicine's way of thinking is to lower cholesterol – the lower, the better – but our knowledge goes way beyond that: we know that cholesterol is essential to and for life, and having a level that is too low is not good – without it we couldn't survive; remember, people whose cholesterol levels drop below 45 mg/dL cannot survive. We also know that cholesterol is not the culprit of arteriosclerosis (hardening of the arteries) and atherosclerosis (plaque in the arteries). So why then should we need to lower it? We don't – we need to normalize it! Meaning, there is a balance between high and low which is normal; neither a too high nor a too low cholesterol level is good. Low cholesterol is the cause of multiple health issues and a crucial factor behind increased mortality rates, specifically because cholesterol is such an important source of many vital agents in the body. Very high cholesterol, on the other hand, is usually a reflection of a profound problem within the mechanism that regulates the production of these vital agents (we will discuss this further later).

However and unfortunately, the statin industry today just keeps pushing the almighty, well-marketed lowering mechanism with no consideration being given to whether it is right or wrong, good or bad. The major way to lower cholesterol is to prescribe a CLD; unfortunately, though, by interfering with a major bodily mechanism that lowers cholesterol levels, it does more harm than good, offering some deleterious side effects. And, of course, it certainly does not resolve heart disease, heart attack or stroke mortality – it may actually increase it.

In truth, what conventional medicine has not yet understood (or maybe it has) is that high cholesterol is an indicator that there is a problem or physiological adaptation going on in the body. There is no smoke without fire! It is smoke that warns us that fire has broken out. Cholesterol-lowering drugs mess with the cholesterol mechanism and lower hormone production along the way, making the situation even worse. Remember, hormones are the single most powerful messaging machine in the human body and are part of what keeps us up and running and the body functioning correctly. CLDs do not put out the fire – they may get rid of the smoke but the underlying fire (root cause) is still burning; it is not being corrected, it is merely being interfered with.

We all know that cholesterol can deposit in the arterial wall and can be a factor in atherosclerotic plaque, which can lead to blockage of the arteries. An initial and superficial glance would suggest that cholesterol needs to be 'got rid of' at this point but, if you remember, cholesterol shows up when there is an injury to the lining of the arteries (fire) – injury caused by free radicals, toxins, infection, etc. – and high cholesterol is the 'indicator' to your problem (smoke). A signal is sent to the liver which then produces the LDL carrier to deliver cholesterol to repair the injury. Once the damage is rectified or repaired, or the enemy is neutralized, cholesterol is shuttled back to the liver in the HDL carrier. Cholesterol is the fireman at work; if we inhibit these fire engines, LDL and HDL, they can no longer do their work, they cannot put out the fire. It makes no sense to interfere with this mechanism.

Dr Dzugan and I have a question for you: if a person were to have a bruise, would it be necessary to drain the body of all its blood just because the presence of blood, in this instance, caused the bruise? No, of course not. Just as with cholesterol, it is the body's natural healing process. Cholesterol should not be cut off at its pass; it is there to protect and heal us.

A Better Understanding of Pharmaceutical Drugs and Their Adverse Reactions

As stated previously, most prescription (chemical) drugs work by blocking receptors or inhibiting (poisoning) desperately needed enzymes – remember, statins work by inhibiting the enzyme HMG-CoA reductase, interrupting cholesterol production and, therefore, hormone production, among other things. In order for the body to function at optimum, it requires the raw materials that are fundamental for the biochemical pathways to produce life-enhancing substances such as hormones, proteins and energy in the form of ATP (adenosine triphosphate – energetic fuel produced in the mitochondria).

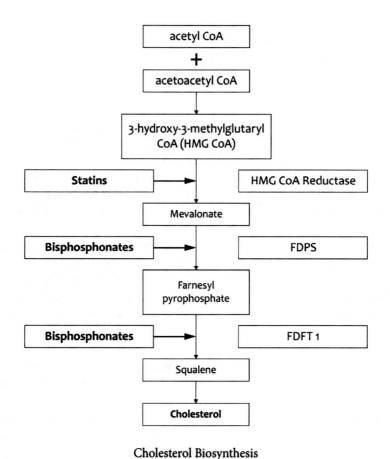

Cholesterol Biosynthesis
(simplified version)

Sergey S. Dzugan, Sergey A. Dzugan. The cumulative effect of biophosphonates and statins on stress fractures. Is it a failure of steroid biosynthesis? Neuroendocrinology Lett (NEL). 2016;37(2):101-5

Understanding these pathways makes it a lot easier to 'figure out' why problems occur when biochemistry is disrupted. The human infrastructure was not set up to have its enzymes poisoned or receptors blocked – they are there for a reason, to work for us, not against us. One does not need a degree in rocket science to understand this – with the long-term use of any drug, we cannot expect a good outcome. These chemical drugs are foreign to the body, they are intruders and set up new reactions which declare war on everything they touch. Of course, there are times when these medications are needed, but relying on drugs that inhibit and poison long term is not a good idea. Many of these drugs can create deleterious adverse reactions, including death.

Bisphosphonates

As an example, let's take a quick look at bisphosphonates which are a chemical drug prescribed to prevent and treat osteoporosis. Although they are meant to treat osteoporosis, recent studies have demonstrated a link between long-term use of these drugs and atraumatic or low-energy atypical femoral fractures.

We have deliberately chosen this drug as an example as it interferes with the mevalonate and squalene pathways, only further downstream to statins, by inhibition of the farnesyl diphosphate. Mevalonate is a vitally important compound that not only furthers the synthesis of cholesterol but also plays an important role in N-glycosylation, which is a specific process related to amino acids, one of which is arginine. Arginine is also a precursor to creatine, and creatine has a vital role in the energy metabolism of muscles, nerves and testes. Another agent on the pathway of conversion is squalene. Squalene plays a significant role in our overall health, having antioxidant properties and, through physiological function, acts as an anti-cancer agent.

Both statins and bisphosphonates have a major impact on the cholesterol biosynthesis pathway and both offer various adverse side effects. Bisphosphonates decrease bone breakdown, interfering with the mechanism between bone breakdown (osteoclast) and renewal (osteoblast). Under normal circumstances, osteoclast and osteoblast live harmoniously together, each balancing the other out. With age and hormonal loss, these two processes become imbalanced. When there is an imbalance between osteoblast and osteoclast activity, two very natural processes, damage to the bone occurs.

Bisphosphonate drugs – the most popular in the US being Boniva (ibandronate), Fosamax (alendronate), and the more recently approved (August 2006) bisphosphonate for male osteoporosis Actonel (risedronate) – all come with risk factors and the possibility of adverse drug reactions. These include: upper-gastrointestinal-tracts adverse events, renal toxicity, ocular adverse events, hypocalcaemia (low blood-calcium level) and secondary hypoparathyroidism (hypoPTH), musculoskeletal pain, osteonecrosis (bone death) of the jaw, arterial fibrillation, atypical fractures related to the thigh bone, and acute phase response such as fever, chills, bone pain, myalgia (muscle pain) and arthralgia (joint pain).

As mentioned previously, these drugs are typically prescribed to prevent and treat osteoporosis – the loss of bone density or the collapsing or 'chalking effect' of bones, which causes kyphosis (excessive curvature of the spine, causing hunching of the back), broken bones, fractures of the spine, and hip fractures. Conventional medicine primarily prescribes these drugs to postmenopausal women who are at a high risk of bone loss due to declining estrogens levels. These drugs are also occasionally prescribed to men, but bone loss in their case is largely connected to the decline of testosterone levels.

Bisphosphonate therapy works by significantly interfering with the cholesterol pathway, and blocking key molecules that are needed for the natural bone renewal and repair process. In other words, bisphosphonates disrupt the physiological mechanism of natural bone repair, meaning, the bone cannot mend itself. Bone is continually renewing and repairing itself (it is a natural and physiological mechanism) and this is how fractures heal. Bisphosphonate therapy suppresses endogenous (natural) bone repair to such an extent that normal bone repair is decreased, leading to a significant increase in 'atypical' fracture risk.

Interfering with the production of cholesterol in any way is not a good idea – remember, cholesterol is needed by every cell in the body to enable it to function correctly and maintain homeostasis. If we don't allow the body what it needs to survive and we interfere with a natural process, danger will ensue and we will definitely have a high rate of adverse drug reactions.

'The Long and Winding Road' of Adverse Drug Reactions

A study done in 1994 which incorporated six major medical centers in the US demonstrated how many adverse reactions happened in hospitalized patients; they also calculated how many hospitalized patients died from adverse reactions to drugs. From these statistics, scientists deduced how many adverse drug reactions took place throughout the US in hospitalized patients. They concluded that over 2.2 million adverse drug reactions resulted in over 106,000 deaths, making these reactions between the fourth and sixth leading cause of death. A lot of people! These deaths occurred not because of their illness but because of an adverse reaction to the medication that was prescribed to and taken by them.

We are now in the 21st century and harm from adverse drug reactions has reached significant numbers. Nearly two decades later, we are being prescribed and are using many more medications which work through the same mechanism (inhibiting enzymes or blocking receptors) than in 1994. It is only obvious, then, that the more medications we take, the more likely we are to suffer from a higher rate of adverse drug reactions.

The Overuse of Pharmaceutical Drugs Today

The abuse and overuse of pharmaceutical drugs today have reached frightening proportions; in the United States, prescription painkillers kill more Americans than heroin and cocaine combined. Individuals taking statins are 87% more likely to develop diabetes. According to the CDC, approximately three-quarters of a million people a year are rushed to emergency rooms in the United States because of adverse reactions to pharmaceutical drugs. And one more: a study conducted by Mayo Clinic showed that nearly 70% of all Americans are on at least one prescription drug, and an incredible 20% of all Americans are taking at least five prescription drugs. Americans spent more than 280 billion dollars on prescription drugs during 2013, and the dollar sign is still going up. Incredible!

The pharmaceutical industries offer us a cover-up drug or a quick fix that doesn't work. These drugs are not a cure! Our doctors can offer us strong blood thinners such as aspirin, a more recently added member Effient (approved in 2009), Plavix, and warfarin (Coumadin). There are medications such as beta blockers, diuretics, angiotensin-converting-enzyme (ACE) inhibitors, calcium-blockers and, of course, statins. None of these drugs work to correct the immediate problem or underlying root cause, they only cover up. And, of course, none of these drugs come without risk or side effects.

The human body has been created with receptors that are set up for natural substances, enabling it to recognize, metabolize and use accordingly. The body has detoxification pathways that remove these natural substances when the body is done with them. This is not true of synthetic substances – the body does not have receptors for synthetic substances. Every time we take a prescription drug, there is a risk of side effects. There is not one single person who would expect these medications to kill them, but they can! It happens far more often than we think.

Generally, natural substances have shorter half-lives than synthetic substances. A half-life is classified as how long it takes the body to rid itself of 50% of the drug. The reason the body has a shorter life for natural substances, compared to synthetic drugs, is because it has receptors for them and understands how to use and dispose of them quickly. Generally speaking, natural substances have a half-life of a few minutes to a few hours. The longer the half-life of a drug is, the greater the risk of adverse effects occurring. Lipitor has a half-life of twenty to thirty hours and Crestor has a half-life of nineteen hours. Of course, this is only one, not the major, problem with statins.

To make an informed decision, whenever any medication is prescribed, we should be aware of the risks at stake – which, of course, need to be weighed against any possible benefits. Whose body is it? Yours! Not your doctor's, not your pharmacist's, it is yours. It is you who has to weigh up the risk factors of your health, your life and/or your death, no one else. It is of paramount importance that you understand your body and therefore your health and how to maintain it.

Understanding Physiological Demand and Cholesterol

Hypercholesterolemia is associated with increased physiologic demand, meaning, those times when the body must prepare itself for a change in function for a particular happening or task.

Pregnancy, Miscarriage and Baby Development Into Adulthood: The Cholesterol Connection

We mentioned previously that cholesterol levels rise to fairly high numbers in pregnancy with no devastating effects on the woman, or baby for that matter. But, remember, when there are diminished levels, a miscarriage may result. It is quite obvious that increased levels of cholesterol are essential for the most optimal and safest fetal development. Another important fact is that, once born, the baby requires adequate amounts of cholesterol for correct neurological development. In fact, that is why breast milk is so rich in cholesterol. The newborn requires cholesterol for optimal neurological and immune function and development. It is building the newborn up, preparing it for a better future. Pregnenolone is the first hormone to be manufactured from cholesterol, which is the precursor to a cascade of other hormones. Pregnenolone is a neurosteroid as well as a steroid hormone. Newborn babies have pregnenolone levels almost ten times higher than those of adults. Pregnenolone is a major neurosteroid required for normal brain development and function.

You will also remember that high levels of cholesterol were seen in up to 53.1% of schoolchildren, which is due to an increased need for anabolic (building) hormones, necessary for growth and physical development into adulthood. Once again, cholesterol is building the human body, not tearing it down.

Stress and the Hormone Connection

Stress, both physical and mental, plays a significant role in increased cholesterol production, which can be attributed to a specific hormone, cortisol, known as the stress hormone. Stress can have devastating effects on the body, one of which is a heart attack. Cortisol production increases in response to any stress in the body (physical and/or mental); it is the body's survival mechanism and is healthy. Cortisol pours when the fight-or-flight situation is engaged but quickly returns to a resting state when the stressful situation is resolved. Interestingly, cortisol has a special relationship with DHEA – both these hormones are produced in the adrenal gland (cortex).

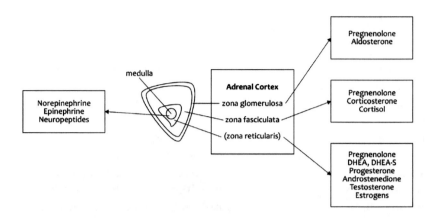

Adrenal Gland

and tearing-down effects are both essential for the body; the levels and ratios of both these hormones must be in balance to counteract each other and to enable us to obtain and maintain optimal health.

The adrenal cortex consists of three zones; all three contain cholesterol, 'the raw material', which is converted into the hormone pregnenolone, which then goes on to make a cascade of other steroid hormones, including progesterone, DHEA, testosterone, estrogens and cortisol.

The special relationship we mentioned previously is known as the cortisol-to-DHEA ratio. The cortisol-to-DHEA ratio decreases when we are calm but increases when we are under acute stress. When cortisol levels are continually high to that of DHEA (something which is known as 'cortisol dominance') due to excessive and long-term stress, the body then requires more cholesterol to balance out disturbed hormone production.

To explain further, when there is long-term stress, cortisol levels will remain high, which will eventually cause the adrenal glands to become damaged or exhausted. This is now a 'chronic-stress situation'. This damage will eventually cause impaired cortisol secretion and regulation which, in turn, will create an imbalance between the two said ratios, bringing with it high, low or normal levels of cortisol.

A chronic-stress situation causes the adrenals to secrete large amounts of cortisol and adrenaline (epinephrine) but, at the same time, the production of DHEA declines. The increased cortisol and adrenaline production will remain high and then will eventually drop to a normal level. The body then tries to adapt to make up for the reduced production of cortisol (in order to cope with stress) and adrenaline by way of a phenomenon called 'pregnenolone steal'. Pregnenolone, DHEA, progesterone, estrogens, testosterone and aldosterone (because pregnenolone is a precursor to all these hormones) then all decline in favor of cortisol. 'Pregnenolone steal' is a stealing process; it is one hormone (cortisol) stealing from another (pregnenolone) to try and adjust the production of another hormone (cortisol) but, in this case, the normally high cortisol compensates by going even higher, which in turn reduces the production of DHEA. The body is always trying to compensate for daily stress but, with long-term stress, it will eventually be unable to secrete adequate levels of cortisol in proportion to the levels of stress. This is when we see a condition known as 'adrenal exhaustion', when cortisol and adrenaline become so depleted that a severe imbalance of the other steroid hormones occurs. Understandably, this whole process involves extra cholesterol production – again, it is a feedback loop mechanism, a physiologic demand.

Immune Response and Cholesterol Increase and Decrease: A Physiological Demand

During immune response and tissue repair, high levels of cholesterol can occur. When there is infection or injury, the body's natural response (defense mechanism) is to produce extra cholesterol to protect the cell membranes as well as our vital organs. Any inflammation in the body can trigger it to secrete excess cholesterol. Cholesterol can be used as a marker of physiological function or dysfunction. As an example, a 2003 study demonstrated that, in critically ill or injured patients, cholesterol levels fell by 33% in the individuals who died, as opposed to a 28% increase in the individuals who survived – the repairman is at work, healing and protecting. Decreased or fixed cholesterol levels suggest that there is a development of infection or organ/metabolic dysfunction. Conversely, an increase in cholesterol suggests organ failure is being resolved. All these examples clearly demonstrate that cholesterol is acting as a body-wide repairman and not as a terrorist.

The Starving Man: Cholesterol Increase and Hormonal Demand

During times of starvation, cholesterol levels increase by 400%, while triglyceride levels decline by 50%. If you remember our earlier discussion on dietary cholesterol and the feedback mechanism, we mentioned that if we eat less cholesterol the liver produces more, and if we eat more cholesterol the liver produces less. In starvation, the increased production of cholesterol can be associated with a greater need for hormones (that are produced from cholesterol) to support and reinforce the body during the loss of a major part of what sustains it (food supply). Again, it is to do with a physiological demand during times in which the body prepares itself for a change in function for a particular task or happening. Cholesterol is working for us, not against us. Triglycerides, which are commonly known as fats, decline because fats store the greatest amount of energy. In times of extreme starvation and when the body has exhausted all the other possibilities of energy support, it will then use triglycerides to obtain its energy output in an effort to keep on surviving. Our body is very well connected and is always trying to protect itself.

Greek Gods and Goddesses and the Hormonal Connection

In times of strenuous physical activity, such as happens with top-class athletes, serum levels of cholesterol increase. This important point, again, can be linked to steroid-hormone production. These Greek gods and goddesses, with their exquisite physiques, cannot build muscle or a 'sculpture-like' body without an increase in anabolic hormone production such as DHEA (dehydroepiandrosterone) and testosterone, whatever weightlifting or fitness program they may be on. A request in hormone production will, in turn, request a rise in cholesterol levels. The body needs more hormones so, to make these hormones, the cholesterol supply too has to increase. The increase may also be due to 'wear and tear' on the muscles – remember, cholesterol is needed for repair.

As you will have understood, whether it be pregnancy, fighting off disease, intense athletic training or starvation, cholesterol acts as a 'protection mechanism'. It is there to heal, to protect, to nurture, to build and improve the human body, not to destroy it.

Before we move any further, let's take a look at the problems related to both high and low cholesterol, helping you to further understand the role of the cholesterol molecule. Like we said, neither high nor low is particularly good – each has its own adverse effects on the body, and it appears that both low and high total cholesterol may be associated with a higher risk of premature death.

An Evaluation of High and Low Cholesterol

Although the emphasis is and always has been on high cholesterol (hypercholesterolemia), primarily because of the association with atherosclerosis, there are many other conditions and effects associated with varying cholesterol levels that should be considered. Whether levels are high or low, and whether the effects are good or bad, they need to be evaluated to better understand human physiology and the demands of the body. Cholesterol is an 'indicator', a marker of our health; it is the builder and protector of our body; it is our repairman and our healer. It is not a rebel of, or terrorist to, the human body.

Mental Function and the Cholesterol Connection

In chapter 2, we mentioned that all cholesterol in the brain is a product of local synthesis. The highest concentrations of cholesterol in the human body are found in the brain. It only makes sense, then, that psychological disturbances may occur when levels are either high or low (not normal). There is a substantial amount of evidence that cholesterol levels are linked to variations in mental state and/or personality. High cholesterol (hypercholesterolemia) has been reported in individuals with schizophrenia, obsessive-compulsive disorder, panic disorder, generalized anxiety disorder and post-traumatic stress disorder (PTSD). On the other hand, children with autism were observed to have decreased levels of total cholesterol.

Low levels of cholesterol have been linked to patients with major depression, dissociative disorder, antisocial personality disorder, borderline personality disorder, and criminal violence. Also, low levels have been associated with suicidal tendencies (attempt and behavior), aggression and impulsivity.

Strokes and the Cholesterol Connection

Yes, what about strokes? We spoke about strokes earlier in the book, both cerebral infarction (ischemic stroke) and cerebral hemorrhage (hemorrhagic stroke). More often than not, major ischemic strokes are seen in patients with lower cholesterol levels. Higher cholesterol levels are associated with minor strokes, and post-stroke mortality is inversely related to cholesterol, meaning, the higher the cholesterol level in a patient, the less likely he/she will die from the stroke. Also, another study involving two groups of patients demonstrated that the group with the lower levels of cholesterol (less than 180 mg/dL) were at a significantly higher risk of mortality due to hemorrhagic stroke, cancer and all causes, as compared to the group with cholesterol levels between 180 mg/dL and 239 mg/dL. In fact, hemorrhagic stroke increased twofold in men when cholesterol levels fell below 160 mg/dL, but higher levels were seen to be protective against cancers in the lung, hematopoietic and lymphatic systems, together with COPD (Chronic Obstructive Pulmonary Disease). COPD is a term for chronic bronchitis and emphysema, which narrow the airways in the lungs.

Coronary Heart Disease (CHD) and the Cholesterol Connection

Elevated cholesterol levels are always associated with coronary heart disease but let's start by saying that, if high or elevated cholesterol levels were the cause of the heart-disease epidemic we see today, then everyone who suffered a heart attack would be walking around with high cholesterol levels. But this is not the case. One particular study, whose purpose was to correlate lipid profile to coronary heart disease (CHD), demonstrated that 70% of patients who had CAD had total cholesterol levels below 200 mg/dL. Another study showed that individuals who had cholesterol levels below 160 mg/dL had a higher rate of death from CHD than those with levels above 240 mg/dL, who had the lowest risk of death. Isn't that the opposite of what conventional medicine is telling us? Another interesting study showed that elevated total cholesterol levels, low HDL and high TC/HDL ratios were not associated with a higher rate of mortality from CHD, hospitalization for heart attacks or all-cause mortality.

Cholesterol and the Cancer Connection

Cancer seems to be well connected to low cholesterol levels. Several prospective studies demonstrated an association between low serum-cholesterol levels and mortality from cancer. Mortality follow-up from a cohort study (a cohort is any group of people who are linked in some way and followed over time) revealed a significant excess of cancer in the lowest decile of serum-cholesterol levels. Another study showed that men with cholesterol levels between 180 mg/dL and 239 mg/dL had the lowest mortality rate but, when levels fell below this range, they had an increased risk of death from cancer or other diseases.

Understanding Cholesterol and Total Mortality

It seems that, with mortality and cholesterol levels, high cholesterol is not as bad as it's been made out to be. Like we said, it is a marker of our health, and our main repairman – an actual hero. However, both high and low levels appear to carry side effects and, as already stated, both appear to be associated with premature death – at this point, what is required is a normal or ideal level of cholesterol.

Further Evaluation: Low Cholesterol Levels

Over the years, the focus has been on lowering cholesterol to absurd and dangerous levels – just take a look at history and where we are today with the new 2013 guidelines. At this point, we should take a closer look at the ever-decreasing baseline of cholesterol and analyze if low cholesterol does actually enhance mortality rates and/or have any good effects at all, for that matter.

When serum-cholesterol levels in hospitalized patients fell below 100 mg/dL, the mortality rate of these hypocholesterolemia (low cholesterol) patients was found to be about tenfold higher than average, demonstrating a strong, linear relationship with serum-cholesterol concentrations. Doesn't look good! To give you another example, in another study, when concentrations of cholesterol were less than 185 mg/dL in men ranging from forty to fifty-nine years of age, it was seen to be associated with the highest mortality rate from all causes.

The Honolulu Heart Program, which was initiated with the study of cardiovascular disease and cholesterol in mind, demonstrated that patients who had lower cholesterol levels than their counterparts had a greater risk of premature death. To explain further, a younger individual with low cholesterol levels will naturally follow 'rule of thumb' and increase cholesterol production with age but, since his cholesterol was lower to begin with, his mortality increases in relation to someone who had the same cholesterol levels but was, let's say, ten years older. Overall, this study showed that caution should be taken with regards to any attempt to lower cholesterol in the elderly.

Overall, cholesterol levels that are below 160 mg/dL are associated with all-cause mortality other than cardiovascular disease, specifically cancer, respiratory and digestive disease, and hemorrhagic stroke. Again in the Honolulu Heart Study, low cholesterol levels were linked to an increased risk of liver disease and cancer but normal or stable levels were not.

Basically, it seems that cholesterol levels should rather be normalized instead of interfered with, enabling optimal functioning of the 'cell signaling setup', else the tightly controlled system will malfunction, resulting in ill health, along with death.

6. A SERIOUS TALK ON STATINS

In chapter 5 we spoke about adverse drug reactions caused by prescription/chemical drugs. Statins, in particular, have been associated with a vast range of adverse reactions. Of course, one could quite easily surmise this, especially knowing that cholesterol is such a vital molecule for every cell in the body and, in fact, every organ system in the body. If you were to starve the body of food over a prolonged period, what would happen? It would cause the body to decrease total body energy expenditure – decreasing metabolic activity as manifested in diminished muscle activity, increased sleep and decreased core temperature. The body would slowly shut down and eventually die. If you starve the cells of the highly needed molecule, cholesterol, the body will dysfunction and premature death will occur. Cholesterol is the building material of the body; we were given this 'almighty' substance but so many of us are unaware of its importance. We need it as we need food to nurture us, to make us strong, to protect us, to repair and heal, and to support and prolong life.

So far, more than fifty adverse effects of statins have been reported to the Food and Drug Administration and we are still counting. The most common adverse effects of CLDs include chest pain, dizziness, weakness, serious fatigue, fibromyalgia, headaches, insomnia and upper-respiratory-tract infections. Other negative side effects include neuropathy (nerve dysfunction), polyneuropathy (pain in more than one nerve), myalgia, cataracts, erectile dysfunction (ED), cognitive impairment/memory loss/dementia/TGA (transient global amnesia), anemia, immune-system suppression, myopathy (muscle weakness and muscle-wasting disease) and cardiomyopathy, kidney failure, pancreatic dysfunction and liver dysfunction. Statins have also been associated with myositis and rhabdomyolysis (a breakdown of muscle fibers) and, the final curtain, death. There is also an increased rate of all-cause mortality, cancer included.

Negative side effects such as lupus-like syndrome, pleurisy, arthralgia, intracerebral hemorrhage, ataxia and cataract have also been documented. Lupus is an autoimmune disease which attacks the body's own tissues;

this can result in inflammation and tissue damage – not a particularly good place to be! Pleurisy is inflammation of the lining of the lungs and chest; this condition can make breathing extremely painful – again, not a good place to be! Arthralgia is a form of arthritis, presenting joint pain but without the swelling. Intracerebral hemorrhage (ICH) is the most devastating type of stroke and occurs when an artery in the brain bursts, causing bleeding into the brain. Importantly, a significant risk of ICH has been observed in people taking a higher-dose statin. Ataxia is a chronic disease of the cerebellum; people with ataxia experience loss of muscle control in their arms and legs, the outcome being a lack of balance and coordination or an abnormal gait. Cataracts cause opacification or clouding of the eye's natural lens, which interferes with visual function; it is the most common cause of vision loss in people over the age of forty and the principal cause of blindness in the world.

Importantly, it should be noted that the myriad of adverse effects offered by CLD were seen in 4%-38% of all patients and resulted in either discontinuation or dose reduction. Also, the occurrence of adverse effects was noted in 73.6% of users of cerivastatin and 74.9% for pravastatin. Another important point to make here is that individuals who began lipid-lowering therapy discontinued it within one year and only about a third of patients reach their treatment goals.

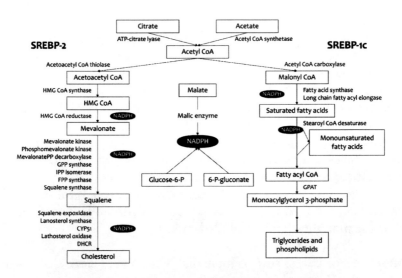

Cholesterol, triglycerides and phospholipids biosynthesis

The Downstream Biochemical Pathways of Cholesterol

In chapter 2 we briefly touched on the biochemical pathways of cholesterol (biochemical pathways are simply a sequence of biochemical reactions controlled by enzymes that help convert molecules or substrates into more readily usable materials). But, if we take a further look at this downstream biosynthetic pathway, we can get a better understanding as to why disturbing cholesterol production, with the use of CLDs, offers so many adverse side effects.

Cholesterol is dependent on the correct functioning of the cholesterol biosynthetic pathway. This pathway is a vital but delicate, tightly controlled and complex downstream process which ensures that each and every cell in the body has an adequate and correct supply of cholesterol. Unfortunately, most of us are unaware of this, including most doctors. It is important to understand this pathway because, if you don't, you cannot possibly begin to understand the importance of cholesterol production and neither can your doctor. The downstream cholesterol pathway is essential for the production of many vital substances, including hormones; if you interfere with this pathway, problems will occur.

The diagram above shows some of the steps required to produce the final product, cholesterol. Remember that a molecule of cholesterol is primarily synthesized or produced from Acetyl CoA through a molecule known as 3-hydroxy-3-methylglutaryl CoA (HMG-CoA). HMG-CoA is then acted upon by an enzyme called HMG-CoA reductase, which eventually goes on to create the final product, cholesterol. Statins work by inhibiting the enzyme HMG-CoA reductase, therefore cutting off cholesterol production, the raw material, in its prime. Importantly, acetyl-CoA is used in many biochemical reactions, including producing the energy molecule adenosine triphosphate (ATP). It is also a precursor for fatty acid, glucose and amino-acid metabolism.

Each step of this pathway is important for normal cell function. Mevalonate stands in the middle of the pathway – mevalonate is the essence of cell renewal; every cell is dependent on mevalonate for its life cycle. In each and every cell, mevalonate travels down the mevalonate pathway to produce cholesterol and isoprenoids (Farnesyl pyrophosphate) (see diagram below). Isoprenoids are produced in both animals and plants. In humans, they are a precursor molecule required for the production of coenzyme Q10 (CoQ-10), dolichols, bile acids and steroid hormones. As we already know, cholesterol-lowering drugs such as statins contaminate the HMG-CoA reductase enzyme, which guarantees a decline in the production of CoQ-10, isoprenoids, bile acids and steroid hormones. A human being cannot live without CoQ-10 and the isoprenoids manufactured in the cholesterol-mevalonate pathway.

Dolichols

As you can see, dolichols are produced further downstream from isoprenoids, following the same intermediate pathway that produces CoQ-10. Dolichols are important molecules for DNA as they carry genetic instructions from the DNA that assist in the creation of specific proteins in the body. With insufficient dolichol production, DNA error can occur due to chaotic and partial messages being relayed, including such problems as cancer. They are vital for glycoprotein synthesis, cell identification, messaging (cell communication), neurohormone formation, as well as immunodefense.

An additional and important point to make here is that dolichols are involved in the manufacture of neuropeptides. Neuropeptides are messenger molecules that send information from the brain to receptor sites found on the cell membranes throughout the body. Until not so long ago, it was thought that neurotransmitters, such as serotonin, GABA (gamma amino butyric acid) and catecholamines (dopamine, norepinephrine, and epinephrine) were the only carriers of information from the brain, assisted by various hormones that traveled through the circulatory system (bloodstream). But we now know that neuropeptides work in harmony with these systems and it is these neuropeptides that transfer the vast majority of information throughout the body. If there is insufficient dolichol production, the entire neurohormone manufacture will then be affected, with devastating results. Although primarily manufactured in the brain, every tissue in the body produces and interchanges neuropeptides, meaning, they regulate nearly all life processes on a cellular level, which goes on to interlink every bodily system. When there is a reduced amount of dolichols, it influences every cellular process in the body; when this process is interrupted, it can have devastating effects on the brain and the body. Neuropeptide regulation is tightly involved with physiology so, when there is a dysregulation of neuropeptide function due to statin use, a host of symptoms can occur, even the most obscure.

Our Behavioral Destiny

Neuropeptides are sometimes known as the 'hormone of emotion' as they can dictate our behavioral destiny. In a complex process of cellular activity, our thoughts, sensations, emotions and, in fact, our very being are clustered together into a tiny chain-like form that 'holds' the ultimate cellular message. Through another complex process, these chain-like peptides are then packaged up and shuttled to their final destination. With insufficient dolichols, the intricate mechanism of neuropeptide formation and transfer cannot successfully occur. As neuropeptides are so involved in emotions and behavior, when there is neuropeptide suppression due to a blockage of mevalonate and, therefore, dolichol production, negative side effects such as personality disruption, depression, irritability, aggressiveness, homicidal behavior, suicide and hostility can result.

Coenzyme Q10 (CoQ-10)

Again, CoQ-10 is produced further downstream from isoprenoid. Statins, as we know, interfere with this vital downstream process by inhibiting the enzyme HMG-CoA reductase, which in turn depletes CoQ-10 production. CoQ-10, also called ubiquinone, meaning 'occurring everywhere', is our most significant essential nutrient and is located in all of our cells. The greatest concentration of CoQ-10 is found in the muscle and, in particular, the heart. The most common adverse drug reaction linked to statin medication occurs in the muscle. In part, the reason statins can cause muscle issues is due to the depletion of CoQ-10. The heart is the largest muscle in the human body and is where, along with the liver, the highest concentration of CoQ-10 is found – both these organs request and require a great deal of energy to perform optimally; with insufficient CoQ-10, heart failure can occur. Knowing that statins inhibit CoQ-10, this should not be surprising and, in fact, the incidence of congestive heart failure (CHF) has tripled since statins first came onto the marketplace. Low levels of CoQ-10 have been implicated in almost all cardiovascular diseases, including angina, hypertension, cardiomyopathy and CHF. CHF happens when the heart muscle is weakened. As a result, the heart cannot pump enough blood and oxygen to the organs and tissues of the body. As the situation worsens, the lungs and extremities begin to fill up with fluid. More than 20 million people are affected by CHF worldwide. According to the American Heart Association, approximately 5.3 million Americans have congestive heart failure (CHF) and approximately 660,000 new cases are diagnosed yearly. CHF is common and is increasing at epidemic rates. Could it be because statins are now so freely and readily prescribed, without giving any thought to the damage they can do? Just something to think about!

Other causes of congestive heart failure are high blood pressure, diabetes and coronary heart disease, and it is also seen to increase in cigarette smokers and obese individuals. However, Dr Dzugan believes that statins are the most overlooked connection to CHF. Remember, the highest concentrations of CoQ-10 are found in the heart, the largest muscle in the body, and statins deplete CoQ-10. Studies show that plasma CoQ-10 concentration is an independent predictor of mortality in individuals with CHF.

CoQ-10 feeds the mitochondria. Mitochondria are the center of our cells and are energy-generating motors. All life functions are dependent on the energetic fuel produced in the mitochondria, known as adenosine triphosphate (ATP). And, in fact, over 90% of the body's energy is produced using CoQ-10 as a cofactor.

Individuals taking Lipitor, the most well-known of statin drugs, have been seen to have up to a 40% decrease of CoQ-10 serum levels. Along with the heart, every cell and every tissue is dependent on the supply of mitochondrial energy. Without sufficient amounts of CoQ-10, our cells lack the appropriate repair mechanism, in other words, they cannot mend or protect themselves.

Apart from assisting in the production of energy, CoQ-10 plays a highly significant role within the mitochondria, acting as a very potent antioxidant, its protective powers against free radicals being fifty times stronger than vitamin E. Free radicals are responsible for disease and breakdown of the body, causing cancers and heart disease. CoQ-10 interacts with many substances in the body such as vitamin C and E, and vitamins B2 and B3, and is an integral and fundamental molecule that feeds muscle cells so that they can produce energy. Any process that depletes CoQ-10 will result in energy and muscle issues.

At this point, one should ask why anyone would manufacture, prescribe or take a drug that kills the enzyme needed to make CoQ-10 and cholesterol for that matter. Beats us!

Extra and Important Information You Need to Know About Statins

Alongside its many vital functions, CoQ-10 also keeps the cell lining elastic. Statins break down cell walls and, as mentioned previously, have been indicated in a condition called neuropathy. Neuropathy is an extremely painful condition characterized by pain, muscle twitching, muscle loss, change in balance and coordination, numbness and tingling. Also, polyneuropathy commonly occurs in long-term statin users. As many as 5,950 cases of neuropathy, 15,580 cases of pain in extremities, 736 cases of coordination problems, and 3,742 cases of balance disorders have been reported by FAERS (FDA Adverse Event Reporting System) between the years 2004 and 2014.

Thought, Memory, Learning, Mental Function: Cognitive Impairment

The brain is a very versatile organ and has a multitude of protective mechanisms in place – interfere with those mechanisms and you will get problems. We know that the highest concentrations of cholesterol in the body are found in the brain and, in particular, the thinking part of the brain, the cortex. The brain cannot function without sufficient cholesterol. It is only obvious, then, that taking a cholesterol-lowering drug will bring with it an increased risk of brain problems and disorders. Adverse effects of statin medication include amnesia (4,720 cases), confusional state (7,171 cases), dementia (1,577 cases), disorientation (2,054 cases), depression (13,290 cases), memory impairment and transient global amnesia (9,004 cases), as well as suicidal ideation, attempt or behavior (3,414 cases), all reported to the FDA from 2004 to 2014.

In chapter 2, we spoke about the myelin sheath. Myelin is a substance that winds around the nerve cell axons. It insulates nerve cells, helps regenerate cut axons and intensifies impulses and electrical messages throughout the nervous system's circuitry. Neuronal communication is not only dependent on cholesterol but the latter is vital. Cholesterol is a fundamental constituent of myelin – when there is loss of the myelin sheath, or demyelination, it has been linked to neurodegenerative disorders such as multiple sclerosis, Guillain-Barre syndrome and demyelinating polyneuropathy. And, in fact, from 2004 to 2014, FAERS reported to the FDA that 1,330 cases of multiple sclerosis, 202 cases of Guillain-Barre syndrome and 334 cases of amyotrophic lateral sclerosis (ALS or Lou Gehrig's disease) occurred due to statin use.

Let's think about this for one second… The myelin sheath is primarily made from cholesterol; it is fair, therefore, to say that anything that interferes with the production of cholesterol will cause loss of the myelin sheath and the demyelination conditions mentioned above, along with other problems. One study found that there was an increased risk of polyneuropathy with statin use and patients who took statins for two or more years had a significantly increased risk of polyneuropathy.

Multiple Sclerosis

Multiple sclerosis is an inflammatory and autoimmune disease whereby the myelin sheath that covers the nerve cells in the central nervous system, involving the brain and spinal cord, becomes damaged. Incredibly, some short-term studies lay claims that statin drugs can be used as a therapy for multiple sclerosis by way of an anti-inflammatory mechanism. Of course, this mechanism is understandable: why wouldn't halting inflammation help? In this case it doesn't! In fact, inflammation is necessary for myelin repair as it stimulates remyelination in areas of chronic demyelination. The truth is, studies show that statins could worsen MS by disrupting the myelin sheath. Statins not only restrict the synthesis of the cholesterol needed for the general health of the myelin sheath, they restrict the synthesis of dolichols (isoprenoids) that are involved in the process of myelin maintenance and remyelination. Statins inhibit and slow myelin repair, leaving the axons unprotected and more exposed to injury.

Amyotrophic Lateral Sclerosis (ALS)

Amyotrophic lateral sclerosis (ALS or Lou Gehrig's disease) is a cruel, slow-moving neurodegenerative illness that involves the nerve cells in the brain and the spinal cord. This horrific disease is characterized by progressive degeneration of motor neurons (that control organs, muscles and glands), which eventually leads to death. ALS has been linked to abnormal lipid metabolism and, in fact, patients with high levels of triglycerides and serum-cholesterol levels have been seen to have a prolonged survival in ALS. As mentioned previously, as many as 334 cases of ALS were reported to the FDA (by FAERS) after having initiated statin medication. Perhaps before prescribing or taking a cholesterol-lowering drug we should think twice! When we inhibit cholesterol, we impair its neuroprotective qualities, among other things. Why take a drug like that, especially since this vital substance, cholesterol, is irrelevant in the atherosclerotic process?

There is no doubt that statin drugs cause neuronal degeneration. If you recall, statins inhibit the production of cholesterol by their effect on the mevalonate pathway. This inhibitory effect on the mevalonate pathway then provokes the induction of abnormal tau-protein phosphorylation, which promotes the formation of neurofibrillatory tangles, long known to be the number-one culprit in the cause of the slow and progressive neuronal degeneration of Alzheimer's disease. This mechanism has also recently been linked to other forms of neurodegenerative disease, including ALS, Parkinson's disease (PD), Frontal Lobe Dementia (FLD) and Multiple System Abnormalities.

Note: Tau proteins are part of a vital cell transport system (a structure known as microtubule), a very well-organized path of parallel strands (something like a railway track). Tau protein strands help maintain cell integrity and assist in the transportation of nutrients within the cells. In other words, they help keep the tracks straight so there is ease of transportation. Inside the cells (neurons) of individuals with Alzheimer's disease, these strands collapse and twist, preventing them from functioning and transporting nutrients and other substances, eventually provoking their death. These are known as neurofibrillary tangles or abnormal tau proteins. We all develop tangles as we age but those with Alzheimer's disease tend to accumulate five to ten times more than normal.

Statin medication has also been linked to the onset of ALS-like conditions, which ameliorate when statin medication is discontinued. Lower serum-lipid levels have also been related to respiratory impairment in patients with ALS.

Parkinson's Disease (PD)

Statins have been associated with a higher risk of PD, whereas higher total cholesterol is associated with a lower risk. In the Atherosclerosis Risk in Communities Study (ARIC), researchers prospectively studied lipid plasma and statin use in relation to Parkinson's disease over a period of eleven years. The authors concluded that: "Statin use may be associated with a higher PD risk, whereas higher total cholesterol may be associated with lower risk. These data are inconsistent with the hypothesis that statins are protective against PD." Another study showed that low levels of LDL cholesterol increase PD risk – remember that LDL levels mirror total cholesterol levels. When one understands the importance of cholesterol and its connection with the optimal functioning of the brain, it should then come as no surprise that the use of statin medication is linked to brain issues such Parkinson's disease. Cholesterol is there to help, not hinder!

Statins and Ataxia

Here we have a fairly new side effect associated with statin use. Ataxia is a chronic disease of the cerebellum which is Latin for 'little brain'. It is the region of the brain that plays an important role in motor control. It also influences some cognitive functions such as language and attention, and plays a role in regulating the fear and pleasure response. However, it is more strongly linked to movement-related functions. People with ataxia experience loss of muscle control in their arms and legs, the outcome being a lack of balance and coordination or an abnormal gait.

Ataxia occurs when parts of the nervous system that control movement become damaged and cells in the cerebellum degenerate or atrophy. Many cases of ataxia are hereditary but acquired or secondary cerebellar ataxia can be caused by conditions such as stroke, multiple sclerosis, tumors, alcoholism, peripheral neuropathy, metabolic disorders and vitamin deficiencies. However, and frighteningly so, a more recent finding shows that progressive cerebellar ataxia can be induced by hydroxyl-3-methylglutaryl-coenzymeA (HMG-CoA) reductase inhibitor – a cholesterol-lowering drug. So, once again, we see neuronal damage and degeneration with the use of statin drugs. Disrupt the cholesterol-producing pathway and we will get 'brain and muscle issues' along the way.

Coenzyme Q10 deficiency has also been linked to cerebellar ataxia. And, in fact, after statin use was withdrawn and a specific treatment with coenzyme Q10 was introduced, progressive improvement of gait ataxia was seen in some patients. If you recall, CoQ-10 is a vital part of the downstream pathway to cholesterol production; it is our most significant essential nutrient and is located in all of our cells.

Myopathy and Rhabdomyolysis

Myopathy, a muscle-wasting disease and a serious condition that can cause congestive heart failure, is often seen in statin users. Remember, the heart is a muscle and statins can impair the pumping functions of the heart. Another outcome associated with CLD use is myositis (inflammation of the muscle) and the deadly rhabdomyolysis. Rhabdomyolysis is the most severe form of myopathy and is a serious condition which involves the breakdown of skeletal muscle tissue. When this happens, there is a release of a protein found in the muscle tissue, called myoglobin, into the bloodstream, which results in myoglobinuria and blockage and damage of the kidneys. Myoglobinuria is when there are large amounts of myoglobin present in the urine, which are usually excreted out of the body. When there is too much of it in the urine, it can affect the filtration mechanism and cause major problems. Myoglobin can also break down into potentially toxic products which then go on to cause kidney failure and, eventually, death. Baycol (cerivastatin), a commonly prescribed cholesterol-lowering drug, was taken off the market in August 2001 because of its association with numerous deaths from rhabdomyolysis. Remember, all statin drugs use the same mechanism: they inhibit the enzyme HMG-CoA reductase. Deaths from this horrific form of muscle-cell breakdown are still being reported.

Note: Although it is well-known that statin users can develop musculoskeletal issues, another important and more recently discovered adverse effect relating to statin use is muscle rupture.

Statins and Diabetes Type 2

If you recall, we touched on statin medication and the diabetes-type-2 connection in chapter 4. Diabetics are often prescribed statins because of their high-risk status of heart attack – diabetes is an independent risk factor for the development of cardiovascular disease. For more than two decades it's been known that statins can adversely affect insulin secretion and sensitivity. And, as we already stated (chapter 4), statins increase the risk of adult-onset type 2 diabetes, with various studies showing that statins can increase the risk by 10%-20%, with the risk being directly linked to the dose of the medication. These particular studies were designed to observe the effects of statins on cholesterol.

The JUPITER trial (an Intervention Trial Evaluating Rosuvastatin) we mentioned in chapter 4 demonstrated, post hoc analysis based on gender, an incredible 50% increase in the incidence of physician-diagnosed diabetes in women who took Rosuvastatin. Also, the Women's Health Initiative (WHI) Study of 153,840 postmenopausal women showed that statins taken for three years demonstrated a significant increased risk of new-onset diabetes.

Another interesting study was done more recently in Scandinavia over a period of six years by a team of six doctors from multiple universities, involving 8,749 non-diabetic individuals. The final results were published on March 4th, 2015 in the medical journal *Diabetologia*, with the study concluding that: "Statin treatment increased the risk of type 2 diabetes by 46%, attributable to decreases in insulin and insulin sensitivity and insulin secretion."

This particular study was specifically designed to observe the long-term effects of statin use with regard to developing type 2 diabetes in otherwise healthy people, rather than just observe the effects of statins on cholesterol over the short term (short-term clinical trials cannot fully describe the risk/benefit of long-term statin therapy). Atorvastatin (Lipitor) and simvastatin (Zocor), the two most common and well-known statins worldwide, were seen to give the worst results. The net positive effect on primary prevention of heart attacks for statins across the board is approximately 10% (and only in those with pre-existing heart disease), so swapping a 10% risk improvement for a 46% risk increase seems incredibly absurd.

Moreover, one particular study done by a set of researchers in Ireland found that there was a categorical lack of evidence to support the use of statin therapy in primary prevention. They also found that statins actually increased cardiovascular risk in women, the young and people with diabetes. Furthermore, statins are linked to triple the risk of coronary artery and aortic artery calcification – coronary artery calcification is the hallmark of potentially lethal heart disease. Why take this drug when it causes so many devastating results and does NOT resolve heart disease? Again, it beats us!

In the Prospective Study of Pravastatin in the Elderly at Risk (Prosper) Trial, a three-year randomized primary and secondary prevention trial involving 5,804 elderly men and women (average age: seventy-six) demonstrated that new-onset diabetes was significantly increased by 30%. Why prescribe statins to the elderly in the first place when cholesterol levels naturally begin to decline at age seventy (see chart below)? And when, in actual fact, high cholesterol levels have been seen to be more protective, at every level, for the elderly – the more adequate the levels are, the longer the lifespan. Everyone over the age of sixty-five should understand that the older you get, the more dangerous it is to have low cholesterol levels. We should take into account that over 90% of cardiovascular events occur in the elderly (individuals over age sixty-five) and almost 48% of American people over the age of seventy-five are now on statin medication.

Many individuals are prescribed lifelong statin therapy; the result of this long-term exposure is extremely important. One study showed that there was a 363% increased risk of diabetes after fifteen to twenty years of statin exposure. The longer you take it, the higher the risk.

Yes, you got it right! Statins increase the risk of diabetes, and the higher the dose, the higher the risk, and the longer the therapy, the greater the risk for everyone who takes them! As we mentioned previously, diabetes is already a risk for heart disease, yet diabetics are continually being recommended high-dose statin therapy to prevent heart disease, usually for life. This just doesn't make sense; why do that?

Interestingly, a recent cohort study showed that short-term statin use in primary prevention was also linked to an increased risk of long-term diabetes and diabetic complications and, we might add, without cardiovascular benefits. There is no getting away from it: it is better to leave statins out of the equation altogether.

Another thing: many longstanding diabetics suffer from peripheral neuropathy, which causes a loss of nerve function, numbness, tingling and pain – statins can make the situation worse. Why prescribe these drugs when it is well known that diabetics suffer from peripheral neuropathy in the first place?

The Cholesterol-Age Axis

Mean Standard Deviation of Cholesterol	
Age	Cholesterol
20-29	188.37
30-39	204.75
40-49	221.43
50-59	232.10
60-69	236.55
70-79	227.53
80+	218.18

As you can see from the above chart, cholesterol levels in the body increase with age until the age of seventy, when they begin to stabilize. Steroid hormones, on the other hand, that are produced from cholesterol, decline with age – keep watching those dots! By the time we reach eighty, cholesterol levels are lower still and comparative to the younger age groups, but without, unfortunately, an increase in the all-so-important steroid-hormone production – remember, hormones are the single most powerful messaging machine in the human body and are what keeps it up and functioning correctly.

Like we just said, almost 50% of American adults aged seventy-five and over are on statin medication. Why? It truly doesn't make sense! Statin therapy is commonly prescribed in the over-eighty-year-old group despite the lack of randomized trial evidence supporting this 'fashion'. Moreover, it has been reported that smoking, hypertension, diabetes, but not lipid parameters, are predictors of all-cause mortality in the elderly.

Statins and Cancer

We already spoke about low cholesterol levels and their association to a higher risk of cancer in chapter 4. To continue, all cholesterol-lowering drugs, from fibrates to statins, have been linked to an increased risk of developing cancer. Remember, these medications all affect the basic mechanism of cholesterol in a major way. Low cholesterol levels are a known risk factor for cancer. In 1996, an article in the *Journal of the American Medical Association* reported that fibrates and statins (the two most popular classes of lipid-lowering drugs) caused cancer in rodents, and often at levels as those prescribed to humans. Admittedly, evidence of cancer and lipid-lowering drugs from clinical trials in humans are inconclusive, largely due to inconsistent results and insufficient long-term studies.

An important note: The Deputy Director for the Division of Metabolism and Endocrine Drug Products for the FDA, Dr Gloria Troendle, noted that the cholesterol-lowering drug gemfibrozil (classed as a fibrate) has repeatedly been shown to increase death rates among users. What Dr Dzugan and I find even more frightening is that Dr Troendle stated that she did not believe the FDA had ever approved a drug for long-term use that was as cancer-causing at human doses as gemfibrozil.

A Good Selling Point: Statins Cure Cancer

There are, of course, studies out there that suggest that there is no association with statins and cancer (of course there is an association, a very big one!) and, strangely enough, there are also studies out there that suggest that statins could be used as an effective anti-cancer drug (ridiculous!) due to their high cytotoxic potency. This simply means being toxic to cells – they kill cells, as does chemotherapy. The principle behind it is the same. This may sound good but it isn't. Yet, we hear you say: "Anything that fights cancer must be good, no?" Not always!

Okay, now you are confused, so let's take a look. Statins break the body down by inhibiting the body's most powerful 'messaging machine', hormones. Remember, hormones are produced from cholesterol and statins inhibit cholesterol. Hormones are the most independent factor for a functional immune system. A major component of having a strong immune system is hormonal health. Hormones communicate with each other, so, when hormones are working in harmony and are balanced, they protect us, in the true sense of the word; hormones protect our hearts, our bones, our brain and our body. When there is a breakdown or disharmony and communication is halted, our body breaks down along with our protector, the immune system, and other body systems. Hormones are what we classify as 'the human network of health'. With a decline or an imbalance of hormones, we cannot expect to be healthy. CLDs create an unhealthy scenario.

So, to continue with this statin and anti-cancer medication theory… The difference between statins and chemotherapy is that statins are used on a daily basis, whereas chemotherapy only lasts as long as it is needed. Whatever, chemotherapy is toxic to our system, to our cells, and is not good. The fact that a statin drug could be potentially used as a chemotherapeutic agent is slightly more than worrying. So, statins kill cells, both cancer cells and healthy cells, as does chemotherapy. But think about this for a second and hang on to that thought – not to be binned! If statins were to be used as an all-over anti-cancer drug and were to be prescribed to people with cancer (or without cancer, for that matter), what would happen? They would duly alter body physiology because statins inhibit cholesterol production, which in turn would cause a decline in hormone production. Hormones play an essential role in supporting the immune system; when hormones are low or become imbalanced, a dangerous scenario will be near at hand. This is when the immune system downgrades or becomes weak, leaving a wide open space for cancer, along with other ailments, to take hold and overwhelm the body – our fight-back mechanism has been disarmed. The thought of chemicalizing the body with these drugs seems absurd. The damage they do, on and at every level, is infinite and tremendously frightening. The thought of destroying the body instead of building it up really makes no sense.

Women and Statins

Both Dr Dzugan and I believe that women are highly underrepresented (but that does not mean to say that men, youth and the elderly are any better represented) when it comes to statin medication, heart disease and total mortality rates. And, in fact, there is not one published trial (with placebo controls) that conclusively establishes that statins reduce mortality in women.

Many people believe that breast cancer kills more women than heart disease. This, of course, is untrue. Heart disease is the leading cause of death for both men and women, although women tend to develop heart disease ten years later than men, post menopause, equaling a man's risk at approximately aged seventy. For this reason, women are now being prescribed statins in ever-increasing numbers. Health professionals are still stuck in 'stuck mode', believing that prescribing statin medication will avoid a heart attack. One would think that, as so many women (and men, for that matter) are now being prescribed CLDs, there would have been clear evidence to show a mortality and cardiovascular mortality benefit. There isn't! Try to remember who is behind these studies Big Pharma! Big profit margins! The more people (both men and women) on statins, the better. The get-rich-quick mechanism!

When studying the use of Crestor in healthy men and women, the JUPITER trial found that there was NO significant reduction in heart attack and death in all participants taking statins compared with the control group (the group that did not take statins). Another primary prevention study and meta-analysis of eight trials looked at the gender benefits of statins in preventing cardio events. In conclusion, the study showed that statin therapy did not reduce the risk of CHD events in women without prior cardiovascular disease, and statins did not reduce the risk of total mortality in either men or women.

Statins reduce neither total mortality nor cardiovascular mortality – remember, dead is dead in any case scenario! A recent study in the journal *Cancer Epidemiology, Biomarkers & Prevention* noted that women who took statin medication for more than a decade had double the risk of developing the two common types of breast cancer: invasive ductal carcinoma (IDC), which starts in the ducts of the breast before spreading inwards and accounts for approximately seven out of ten breast cancers cases, and invasive lobular carcinoma.

Experts at the Fred Hutchinson Cancer Research Center in Seattle, USA, also found that the possibility of contracting invasive lobular carcinoma, accounting for 10%-15% of breast cancers, went up almost 2.5 times in some women on statins long term.

Also, the use of statins, in particular lipophilic statins (fat soluble), was linked to an increase in the non-melanoma-skin-cancer (NMSC) risk in post-menopausal women in the WHI (Women's Health Initiative) study cohort.

The reasoning behind this is, of course, hormonal disruption. Statins affect hormone regulation in the body, they stop the cholesterol-production mechanism and, therefore, interfere with hormone production. Interfering with hormone production will cause an imbalance of hormones. It is only obvious, then, that women on statin medication are significantly more likely to suffer from estrogen-sensitive cancers. Remember, hormones are the 'human network of health' and are also the most independent factor for a functional immune system.

We are asking, why on earth, then, would anyone take a statin drug, especially when it can cause cancer, increases total mortality, and does not resolve coronary heart disease?

7. AN ACCURATE ACCOUNT: RESTORATIVE VERSUS CONVENTIONAL MEDICINE

At the beginning of this book, we touched on restorative medicine and how it was based on solid scientific research and evidence. It is now time to take a deeper look and understand what restorative medicine truly is and how it can help you achieve normalized cholesterol levels, which is key to optimal body function, and thus avoid cholesterol-lowering drugs. At the same time, it can enable you to achieve optimal health, a disease-free life, along with positive longevity. It is about maintaining confidence, memory, competence, vitality, positivity, mobility, libido, vision and the foresight you had in your youth until the very end of life. This is possible.

Restorative medicine is a complete medicine, a real medicine, a medicine that considers and treats the body as a whole. It's a medicine that wants to treat you to stay healthy and wants to prevent you from ever becoming ill. It is a medicine that doesn't wait for your body to be so broken and sick that it can no longer be treated – that's the old approach; that's conventional medicine's approach.

Restorative medicine views the body and health in a complete sense – it is a 'whole-body approach'. Optimal health (optimal body function equals optimal health) is what restorative medicine is looking to achieve: the hormonal network, along with internal organs and systems, functioning at maximum efficiency. Restorative medicine looks at prevention, not only cure, by keeping the body totally and optimally balanced. The real goal is to restore function and not necessarily treat disease; it wants to maintain or correct function before illness has a chance to silently but surely creep in. This is the essence of restorative medicine. Restorative medicine is for everyone; you don't have to wait for the body to go into 'physiological breakdown mode' before searching for a qualified restorative doctor. Better sooner than later.

Restorative medicine addresses physiological breakdown and corrects physiological errors we acquire with age by optimizing our physiological profile. Cholesterol levels, for example, that naturally increase with age are due to an age-related decline in endogenous (manufactured in the body) hormone production. This is a clear sign that something is malfunctioning within the body; it is a warning sign. This is what is known as physiological error. This is what is classed as a symptom: your body is talking to you, telling you something is wrong. Symptoms are the body's way of trying to regain homeostasis (balance): your body's defense mechanism.

Restorative medicine offers us something unique: life. It extends our life-span, together with prolonging youth-span and health-span, through early detection, prevention, treatment and reversal of age-related dysfunction, disorders and diseases in both men and women. This is a branch of medicine that strengthens the immune system, rebuilds and restores the body, correcting hormone imbalances with the use of bioidentical hormones (hormones that have the same molecular structure as substances produced in the body), vitamins and minerals, which all interact to enhance and optimize body function, naturally and gently restoring the vitality, energy and vigor of your youth without any harmful side effects. If you recall (chapter 6), we stated that hormones are the most powerful 'messaging machine' in the human body and are the most independent factor for a functional immune system. A major component of having a strong immune system is hormonal health – hormones are, remember, 'the human network of health'. When hormones are balanced, they protect us; when there is a decline, an imbalance or disharmony, the body breaks down along with our protector, the immune system, and other bodily systems.

Bioidentical hormone therapy restores harmony, stability and balance throughout the body, its systems, the mind and emotions, offering an amazing opportunity to live a long and healthy, disease-free life. We have become used to accepting the aging process as normal – becoming ill, frail, weak, tired, being overweight, having cholesterol levels that are not within normal or adequate ranges, having diabetes, etc. It doesn't have to be like that. We have become used to hearing about friends and neighbors dying from cancers, heart disease and Alzheimer's (the three major killers) every other day. We are used to hearing that more than half of the Western world over fifty is, or should be, according to conventional medicine, on a statin drug with the intent to lower cholesterol and supposedly cure heart disease. We know it doesn't cure heart disease it only makes the situation worse by offering us a myriad of health issues!

Bioidentical hormones are the present and the future, a safe alternative and are so much better than the cancer-causing synthetic hormones of bygone days. They are far more efficient, effective and functional than any drug, statins included, on the marketplace today. Bioidentical hormones are life-giving hormones. With a small commitment to enhancing your lifestyle and supported by these life-giving hormones, you can extend your life and the pleasures that go with it by decades, along with normalizing your cholesterol levels. And – again, we repeat ourselves – without any form of cholesterol-lowering drugs which, if you recall, have a high risk of mortality from any cause and offer many deleterious side effects. An optimal state of health and wellness can be achieved at any age; normalized cholesterol levels are intricately entwined in that optimal health scenario. If cholesterol levels are not within a specific ratio (balanced, neither too high nor too low) for the individual, then optimal health will remain elusive. The effects of aging, ill health and this obsession with these dangerous cholesterol-lowering drugs no longer need to be tolerated. Cholesterol levels that are not within normal ranges can now be corrected – no statin drugs involved. You can enjoy your life whether you are 'fifty plus' or younger, without the fear of being told that you have to take a CLD. Instead, you can rebalance your life so that you have a deeper inner silence, relaxed peace, regenerated enthusiasm for life and sex alike, enhanced vitality and boosted positivity, together with total health, enabling you to live life well into your golden years and enjoy infinite wellness. Absolutely no pharmaceutical drugs involved.

We must add, though, that restorative medicine is not about being obsessed with youth; it is about being healthy until the very end of life. It is about protecting and enhancing your maturing health. It is about being proactive about the aging process, taking care of yourself so that you can live the life you want to, not the life that has now become the expected norm of illness and disease, debilitating or otherwise – this, unfortunately, is what conventional medicine has to offer. We no longer have to settle for subpar health; restorative medicine can offer us so much more. Life is about enjoying every stage of it, being able to embrace the experiences and lessons learned and using them to the full until the very end. Restorative medicine aids us in aging with style, grace, vibrancy and energy, maintaining that easy movement, clarity of thinking, sexuality, sensuality and zest for life we had in our youth. Each stage of life is wonderful when you are truly well. It is utterly disastrous to think that so many people will live their later years in ill health, misery and solitude, thwarted by a dysfunctional body and mind, drowning in a sea of despair and pain, a life of endless medical appointments and chemical drugs to treat totally preventable disorders such as high/low cholesterol levels and a lot more. There is an alternative to this dark and frightening scenario – restorative medicine is the answer.

This, of course, is not to say that conventional medicine does not have a place in this world, because it does. However, it should be used as a last resort and, without doubt, cholesterol-lowering drugs should be struck from the marketplace altogether. Conventional medicine has given us many important things: surgery and anesthetic, blood transfusions, and penicillin and other antibiotics that have changed the world forever. These drugs have expanded the human lifespan greatly over the decades but, unfortunately, not always the quality of it. Any chemical drug, including and especially cholesterol-lowering drugs, sets up new reactions that declare war on everything they touch. More often than not, lifetime drugs cause problems and adverse side effects to another part of the body, which then need to be corrected by another form of drug and so it goes on until we get weaker and weaker, sicker and sicker. Drugs do not heal, they only abate. Drugs do not get to the root cause, they only cover up, something like a Band-Aid, until another health issue occurs that is perhaps much more serious.

Restorative medicine, on the other hand, discovers the root cause and corrects it instead of suppressing and hiding those niggling ailments and symptoms which will, at a later date, become something more serious. Restorative medicine focuses on the symptoms, identifies the underlying cause and corrects it. It focuses on YOU, the patient. Restorative medicine is the only thing that can normalize cholesterol levels without any adverse side effects, ward off illness, fatigue, migraine, weight gain, depression and, at the same time, protect against heart disease, cancers, diabetes, Alzheimer's and many other chronic diseases.

Remember to Educate Yourself: Forewarned Is Forearmed

Where health is concerned, there is no better way than to educate yourself – knowledge is power. In today's society, the scope and complexity of chronic disease and medical conditions that are so prevalent are not only heartbreaking but also breathtaking: Crohn's disease, ulcerative colitis, fibromyalgia, lupus, multiple sclerosis, migraine, chronic-fatigue syndrome, osteoporosis, as well as the above-mentioned. More often than not, the treatment recommended by conventional medicine is so toxic that it is worse than the actual illness. Just take a look at individuals who have been on long-term synthetic steroids that supposedly treat some of these conditions: these synthetic steroids tear your immune system down, they kill it, allowing diseases such as cancer and many other devastating illnesses to take hold. Bioidentical hormones, on the other hand, activate, enhance, regenerate and strengthen the immune system, helping to hold chronic disease and cancers at bay, promoting the healing and repair process in the body along the way. To successfully treat any disease, it is important to understand the underlying cause of that particular illness. It is impossible to develop an effective treatment until you know what the underlying cause is and where it is coming from; conventional medicine does not get this – restorative medicine does! Understanding restorative medicine is understanding that the majority of chronic illnesses is due to a hormonal imbalance.

It is truly important that the layperson becomes aware of the treatment options available. Patients, in particular, should educate themselves about the prescription drugs they are taking and investigate natural alternatives such as restorative medicine. In that way, they will be better prepared when making healthcare decisions.

What Are Bioidentical Hormones and Synthetic Hormones (Conventional Hormones)?

Bioidentical hormones have been available since the 1930s and are considered a natural component – they are not a pharmaceutical drug. These plant-based supplements are compounded from plant extracts, such as soy and wild yam, that are then bioengineered in a lab to become an exact copy of the human hormone. A good example is manmade progesterone that is synthesized in a laboratory from the molecule of so-called diosgenin, found in wild yam, giving a molecule-identical result. Wild yam does not contain progesterone so, to achieve a natural-progesterone result, it has to be made in the laboratory. This ensures that the progesterone is one hundred percent bioidentical or natural to the requirements of the human body.

These are life-giving molecules and protect us in various ways by restoring hormone levels that naturally decline with age, preventing a host of health issues and innumerable diseases. A steady decline of critical and vital hormones will eventually lead to an array of complex and debilitating health issues.

As bioidentical hormones are exactly the same in terms of molecular structure, our bodies know exactly how to take these natural substances and metabolize them in precisely the same way they metabolize the body's natural hormones, using them for energy, repair and regeneration, and excreting them when necessary and without difficulty. They cause no known harmful side effects when prescribed correctly. The research and use of bioidentical hormones has been well-documented for many years but it is only in the last decade that they have become more widespread and known to the general public. Bioidentical hormones, when prescribed in physiological not pharmacological doses, are the pathway to optimal health. These unique molecules interconnect to activate every system in the body, aiding the mind-body connection of optimal health.

Note: A physiological dose refers to a dosage required to maintain normal or optimal levels of hormones. These are doses small enough not to cause problems within the body. When doses are too high, as occurs in pharmacological doses, the body will then shut down the production of its own hormones. The body senses that there is too much of the hormone in circulation. When hormones are prescribed in physiological doses, this doesn't occur. When pharmacological doses are used, the body then becomes dependent on those larger doses and negative side effects will occur.

A very important distinction needs to be made between bioidentical hormones and synthetic hormones (produced by the pharmaceutical establishments): bioidentical hormones are safe and effective for the reasons stated above and come without the risks linked to synthetic hormones; synthetic hormones, on the other hand, are concocted from potentially harmful ingredients, such as pregnant mare's urine (synthetic estrogens) and progestins (synthetic progesterone such as Provera), as seen in hormone replacement therapy (HRT) and the contraceptive pill. As these hormones are a non-natural substance, the body cannot metabolize these alien hormones safely and efficiently without going on to produce toxic by-products which will eventually create a drastic situation in the body, including cancer. We believe a more precise term for HRT would be 'hormone substitute therapy' rather than 'hormone replacement therapy', primarily because women's natural hormones are being 'substituted' (definitely not replaced) with a chemical drug. How can you possibly replace something in the body that has never existed in the body something the body has never had? Drugs like these do NOT belong in the body. They are not a replica of our own hormones, they are similar yet different and therefore act differently in the body. The pharmaceutical industry takes natural molecules and tweaks them so that they can be patented (patented pharmaceuticals make money, lots of money).

Chemically altering by adding or subtracting one or two atoms of a molecule, for example, makes a big difference to how the body is affected; even very small amounts can create major effects. For example, the difference between testosterone and estradiol (a type of estrogen) is only one hydrogen atom and a couple of double bonds. Now, just imagine what pharmaceutical companies do to perfectly natural hormones when they add whole chains of molecules and what effect these have on our bodies. They are not making a drug that works better but, by doing so, they are inventing one that behaves similarly yet differently enough to be patentable, one that does us more damage in the long run.

Natural Hormone	A Drug
The progesterone in your body (endogenous)	A drug (progestin) used to replace progesterone in your body

The truth is that the body has an inbuilt system that metabolizes our own hormones and, therefore, natural bioidentical hormones easily and efficiently. For every natural hormone there are enzymes and other chemicals that work exclusively to produce a smooth, non-problematic, no adverse-side-effect landing. And, in fact, estradiol that is produced in the body is easily eliminated through urine within one day, while the synthetic form (Premarin), as used in HRT, can take up to weeks or more post-treatment, due to storage and slow release from fat (adipose) tissue. The body does not want or need these synthetic hormones; they confuse the mind and body setup, provoking a dangerous situation. The human body is, in fact, designed to metabolize endogenous estrogens (and all endogenous hormones) or, in this case, bioidentical hormones that are an exact copy of our own, NOT horse hormones. Chemically created hormones do not belong in the body. The body does not have a deficiency of these synthetic hormones and never will do.

Synthetic hormones are extremely problematic to the body. One of the major issues with progestins (synthetic hormones), versus bioidentical progesterone, is cancer. Women who use the conjugated form of horse estrogens and progestin (HRT) have a significant increased risk of breast cancer, while women who use bioidentical progesterone have a significant decrease in breast cancer risk.

What is Optimal Health?

At the beginning of this chapter, we established that restorative medicine's overall goal is to achieve optimal health. To achieve this, we need to obtain optimal hormone levels, each balanced perfectly and within the correct ratios, so as to mimic our healthiest prime. It is absolutely impossible to achieve optimal health without first accomplishing balance within the hormonal system. Every system in the body – including the cardiovascular system, the nervous system, the circulatory system and the immune system – is dependent upon a balanced hormonal system.

Optimal hormone levels are the key factor to overall health, in normalizing cholesterol levels and sustaining longevity. When we say optimal levels we mean the optimal levels that you had when you were young. At about aged twenty-five, our hormone levels are at their peak and, therefore, this is when we are at our best, both mentally and physically. This is why restorative medicine uses these levels as a guide in achieving optimal health. Thereafter, hormone levels slowly decline, the decline accelerating as time goes on. The objective is to restore hormone levels to a youthful, healthy, energetic level. Importantly, though, we need the correct amount, neither too much, nor too little – we need to find balance. This can only be achieved by an expert in restorative medicine. Restorative medicine is an art. It is a real medicine and one that works.

To ensure robust health and a strong and vigorous future, declining hormones need to be restored. Otherwise, the body will be unable to function optimally and the 'body-breakdown' process will continue to slide into the depths of despair.

8. HORMONES FOR HEALTH (NOT FOR DISEASE)

In chapter 6, we discussed the biosynthetic pathways for the creation of cholesterol and the multiple processes that occur in this pathway, along with the blockage, by way of a cholesterol-lowering drug, of the enzyme HMG-CoA that is necessary for the production of cholesterol, the final product, before going on to be converted into a cascade of steroid hormones. Therefore, CLDs do the job they were designed to do, i.e. lower cholesterol but they do not, we might add, resolve the problem of heart disease.

So What Have Hormones Got to Do with It Then?

Let's start by saying that anything that inhibits cholesterol will interfere with hormone production. Hormones are essential for the correct functioning of the human body and physiology – our hormones are a key component to our overall health. It is, therefore, important to understand the role steroid hormones play within the body, in total wellness and in longevity. Understanding hormone synthesis will, once again, help you to understand the delicate and tightly controlled mechanism in the body. Interfere with any bodily system and you will create an unnecessary 'time bomb' of ill health.

At this point we feel we should emphasize that drug companies know only too well that when cholesterol production is suppressed, steroidal production will also be suppressed. However, these conniving, money-making drug companies deliberately cover this fact up by sponsoring studies that demonstrate that, of course, CLDs have no major effect on steroid-hormone production. If it were proven that CLDs did, in fact, impact steroid-hormone production, these drugs would have an even bigger question mark hanging over their heads. This would be the evidence, without a shadow of a doubt, that these drugs can, in fact, cause drastic and dangerous downstream effects on physiology.

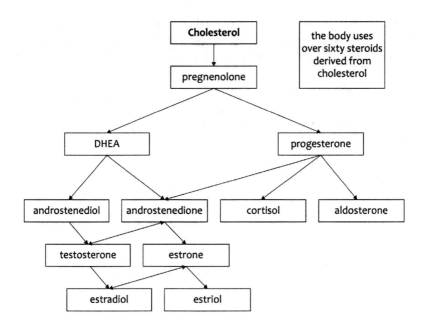

Metabolism of Cholesterol
(simplified version)

The hormonal system, which is commonly known as the endocrine system, controls many important physiological functions in the body. The foundation of the endocrine system is the hormones and glands. Most of the body's hormones are produced by the glands of the endocrine system. These glands include the hypothalamus, pituitary gland, pineal, thyroid and parathyroid glands, adrenal glands, pancreas, ovaries and testes.

The word 'hormone' comes from the Greek language and means 'to set in motion', which is very appropriate as our hormones are shifting all the time in an effort to maintain harmony within the body. Everyone's hormones are as unique as a fingerprint and our DNA.

Hormone levels consistently change or shift throughout life; the amount of hormones the body manufactures and the degree to which they fluctuate or change are important factors in how our body functions or dysfunctions. There are many factors that influence hormonal production: age is one (a big one), stress is another, others are toxins, taking antibiotics, an unhealthy diet, too little or too much exercise, taking too many vitamins or too few and, of course, cholesterol-lowering drugs, alongside bisphosphonates that we mentioned previously in chapter 5 and other conventional drugs.

The key point to keep in mind is that hormones decline with age; this becomes slowly evident at the age of thirty, shifting into second gear at forty, then third gear at fifty, accelerating into fourth and fifth as time goes on. This goes hand in hand with the fact that we are genetically programmed to die.

Why is it, then, that we don't all die at the same age? Why not all die at aged eighty or eighty-one if it is this hormonal decline that dictates our natural death? Good question! Or why don't we all have the same health issues and impairments due to this decreased hormone production? Another good question! It is because we are all different, we all regulate, metabolize and use hormones differently. And, of course, we all lead different lifestyles. There is not one individual that is the same as the other; we all function differently.

The Great Regulators and Controllers

Hormones decline because the endocrine glands cannot keep up the same production of hormones as we made in our younger years. Hormones affect every bodily process and have an enormous influence on the way we look and feel. They are vital for repair and are the most powerful molecule in the regulation of an optimal physiology. They are vital parts of the neuro-endocrine-immune system. The neuro-endocrine-immune system simply refers to three major systems. The nervous system is a collection of all the neurons in the body that are responsible for transmitting impulses and signals throughout the body. There are various subdivisions of the nervous system, such as the central nervous system which includes the brain and spinal cord, and the peripheral nervous system which includes the sympathetic and parasympathetic systems. However, it is the endocrine system that is more directly linked to the production of hormones as it is directly in charge of manufacturing a vast and varied amount of hormones through the aforementioned glands.

Hormones transport information from the brain to the glands, then from the glands to all the cells throughout the body, and from the cells to the brain. In cells, hormones control cell proliferation, differentiation (a process by which cells become more specialized cells), protein synthesis, metabolic rate, etc. Basically, a hormone is a chemical substance produced or secreted by the gland. Hormones are the body's chemical messenger that sends instructions or information from one set of cells to another. No less than 60 trillion cells are affected to a certain degree by these extraordinary hormones. From the moment the umbilical cord is cut and our first breath is taken, hormones are key to how we function, grow and age.

How it works: the glands of the endocrine system release important hormones – such as pregnenolone, estrogens, testosterone, progesterone, DHEA, cortisol, aldosterone, melatonin and thyroid hormones – directly into the bloodstream and then search out cells fitted with special receptors. The release of these hormones is controlled by a master gland in the brain called the hypothalamus. Their goal is to reach their specific destination; each specific hormone is designed to deliver specific information to a specific cell group or organ throughout the body. Once the hormone has been recognized, metabolized and used, it then travels to the liver to be broken down and expelled from the body. If just one part of this process fails, a hormonal imbalance will occur.

Hormones talk to each other, they network and are all interrelated, mutually pumping each other up or slowing each other down to achieve homeostasis. Homeostasis is simply described as equilibrium or balance which is maintained by various feedback mechanisms, both positive and negative. A very simple example of homeostasis is the regulation of our body temperature or the acidity or alkalinity (pH) of our blood.

Hormones are players of a team that is responsible for the maintenance of our health. Block the manufacturing plant, cholesterol, by taking a statin drug and we disrupt our hormone production; mute our cholesterol production and we mute our hormone production. Mute our hormone production and we take away our health. It's as simple as that! Remember, hormones are the 'human network of health'. With low or declining hormone levels we cannot expect to be healthy or stay healthy.

The Endocrine Glands and Hormonal Genesis

The hypothalamus plays a role in growth, appetite, conversion of food into energy (metabolism), blood pressure, our level of sexual activity, our mood, and our responses to heat and cold. It is the major link between the endocrine system and the nervous system. These two systems are the most profoundly affected by regulation – regulation means that the organs and tissues are able to respond appropriately to a stimulus: they understand the message. Each system has a feedback on the other and works in harmony when functioning at optimum. The nervous system works at breakneck speed, regulating within seconds; the endocrine system, on the other hand, functions more slowly, its adjustments taking from minutes to hours to develop.

The hypothalamus is often called the hormone receptionist, receiving messages that come from the brain, which in turn release hormonal messages to the pituitary gland located just below the hypothalamus. It is the keeper of internal balance and homeostasis, and acts as a call center for most of the body's hormonal systems.

Pituitary Gland

The pituitary gland is located at the base of the brain and is about the size of a pea. It is divided into two distinct parts – the anterior and posterior lobes – and produces hormones that control several endocrine glands, each part producing specific hormones when prompted by the hypothalamus. The pituitary gland produces hormones that are essential in maintaining homeostasis in the body. As with all endocrine glands, the hormones that are produced by the pituitary gland are released into the bloodstream and then go on to stimulate target glands – such as the thyroid, adrenal and reproductive glands – to secrete their specific hormones. The target glands respond to the specific hormone as they bear receptors for that specific hormone. In other words, receptors bind to the given cell membrane or organ (which is genetically programmed) like a key in a lock to produce the requested effect on the metabolism and function of the target organ.

Pineal Gland

The pineal gland is a pine-shaped gland, hence its name, and is about the size of a raisin. It is located deep in the brain where it is lodged in a tiny cave behind the ocular nerves. It communicates closely with the hypothalamus to help govern various biological rhythms; it is the body's timekeeper and knows our age. The pineal gland is photosensitive, meaning, it is activated by light. The retinas of the eyes send information or communicate through the sympathetic nerve system to the pineal gland, which then translates these impulses to release certain hormones in the brain. The pineal gland's primary function is to produce and secrete the hormone melatonin. Melatonin is the hormone that is linked to the sleep-wake circadian (daily) cycle.

Adrenal Glands

If you recall, in chapter 5 we discussed the adrenal glands, the inner (medulla) and outer (cortex) regions. Each region produces its own specific hormones: the cortex is responsible for corticosteroids, whereas the medulla is responsible for catecholamines (epinephrine and norepinephrine), and each has very different yet important functions.

The adrenal cortex consists of three zones; all three contain cholesterol, which is converted into the hormone pregnenolone. Remember, pregnenolone goes on to produce a cascade of other steroid hormones, including DHEA, progesterone, cortisol, estrogens and testosterone.

Zona glomerulosa produces aldosterone and pregnenolone and helps maintain blood volume and pressure by way of controlling the blood balance of sodium to potassium.

Zona fasciculata produces cortisol (the stress hormone) and pregnenolone.

Zona reticularis produces pregnenolone, progesterone, DHEA and DHEA-S, as well as a small amount of estrogens and testosterone – although the latter two hormones are mainly produced by the ovaries and testes. After menopause, all women's sex hormones are made by the adrenal glands.

Males' adrenals are usually slightly heavier than those of females. The adrenal glands are strategically placed near the aorta, which is the major artery of the body, and the major vein called the vena cava. This allows for a very rapid response to hormonal messages relayed through the bloodstream. Also, the adrenals are placed in near proximity to the liver, pancreas, major fat storage areas and the kidneys. These organs require rapid and immediate communication with the adrenal hormones. The wisdom of the human body!

The adrenals' hormones are prompted by the hypothalamus and then go on to communicate with the pituitary gland. The pituitary gland then communicates with the thyroid and back to the adrenals. This is a vital communication network in the body – break it and you break the human infrastructure that assists in keeping you healthy. Because of this so-called loop, the adrenals talk to all the other hormones and guide them. The adrenals direct the rest of the endocrine system to keep all the hormones balanced and are very important, in fact, critical, in the building up or breaking down of our health. If cholesterol is disturbed, blocked or inhibited in any way, then it is only obvious that the production plant cannot work efficiently. Hormones will not be produced in sufficient quantities, which in turn will cause a breakdown of the human body and consequently a host of health issues. It is impossible to be healthy without correctly functioning hormonal systems and, for the hormonal systems to operate correctly, all the endocrine glands (adrenal, pituitary, thyroid, ovaries and testes) must be working at full capacity and at their respective optimal levels. Cholesterol-lowering drugs inhibit this delicate 'total-body' mechanism.

The Ovaries and Testes

The ovaries and the testes are more well-known by almost everyone so need little explanation. Ovaries are responsible for the production of estrogens and progesterone which are known as the 'female' hormones, even though men have these hormones as well, albeit at different levels. Women have higher levels of estrogens and progesterone, whereas men have lower levels. The testes are responsible for the production of testosterone, which is known as the 'male' hormone, even if women have this hormone too. Men have higher levels of testosterone, whereas women have lower levels. It goes without saying that both ovaries and testes are vital for reproduction. We will go over estrogens, progesterone and testosterone in more detail later, as well as the important, vital and various roles they play in the body, apart from their reproductive duties.

The Pancreas

The pancreas is about the size of a hand and is found in the upper abdomen, lying behind the stomach and the intestines (gut). The pancreas is important both for hormones and digestion. The pancreas has a connection to the duodenum, which is the first part of the gut, and is connected to the stomach via a tube or duct. This duct allows the digestive enzymes that are made by the cells in the pancreas to travel to the small intestine to help break down agents such as carbohydrates, lipids and proteins, which in turn helps the intestines to absorb these nutrients. About 90% of the pancreas is dedicated to making digestive enzymes. Enzymes are special chemicals which speed up the body's processes. The pancreas also secretes hormones; approximately 5% of the pancreas produces hormones. The hormones made in the pancreas are produced by several different cells which cluster together to form little islands or islets within the pancreas. These islets are known as islets of Langerhans, of which there are about one million dotted around the adult pancreas. The two main hormones secreted by the cells in the islets of Langerhans within the pancreas are insulin and glucagon. Insulin is responsible for lowering blood glucose, while glucagon is responsible for increasing blood glucose. Therefore, it is quite obvious that the correct functioning of the pancreas is important to avoid diabetes, among other things. Other hormones made by the cells in the islets of Langerhans include somatostatin, which helps control the release of other hormones, and gastrin, which aids digestion in the stomach.

Thyroid Gland

The thyroid gland, more commonly known as the thyroid, is a very significant gland and the largest in the human body. It is found in the lower part of the neck, just below the Adam's apple, and releases the iodine-containing hormones thyroxine (T4) and triiodothyronine (T3). Iodine is acquired through food intake. This gland regulates the body's metabolism, temperature and heart rate. Functions of the thyroid gland include: tissue repair and development, aiding the function of mitochondria, controlling hormone excretion, controlling oxygen utilization, regulating vitamin usage, assisting in the digestion process, regulating growth and stimulating protein synthesis.

Thyroid function is very complex and profoundly affects nearly every other organ in the body, therefore the body and its systems are dependent on the correct functioning of the thyroid gland. The thyroid gland is under the control of the pituitary gland, which directly tells it how much thyroid to produce by creating a thyroid-stimulating hormone of its own (TSH). All cells in the body communicate with each other and every cell in the body is affected by the thyroid as it controls the speed at which energy is used by the cells.

Knowledge Is Power!

By now you will have understood that the glands of the endocrine system are, in fact, production plants manufacturing important hormones that all interact with each other, communicating with one another in an effort to maintain homeostasis which, in turn, maintains health. When this team is not functioning correctly, or working in concert, the body will shift into a state of imbalance or 'breakdown' mode. When there is an imbalance of even just one hormone, it will go on to affect the efficiency of the other hormones – the communication system is now down, which will provoke a breakdown of the human infrastructure and, therefore, our health. We cannot expect to be or stay healthy under these circumstances. These production plants, or glands, need the raw material to undergo the lengthy and complex process for the creation of these steroid hormones. Cholesterol is the raw material or molecule from which these steroid hormones are made. Without cholesterol, the body breaks down and begins to dysfunction, bringing with it a myriad of health problems. It is cholesterol that dictates our health. This is what is called physiology of the human body. Without optimal physiology we cannot have optimal health. Without cholesterol we can have neither of these. We cannot party!

Time to Talk Hormones

Pregnenolone

We know that hormones decline with age, and pregnenolone is just one such example. At aged seventy-five, we have approximately 65% less pregnenolone than we had when we were thirty-five. Pregnenolone is what we like to call a 'top-of-the-range' hormone and is a direct descendent of cholesterol. It is the precursor hormone for the adrenal and sex hormones and is often referred to as the 'grandmother hormone' – all the adrenal and sex hormones are produced downstream from pregnenolone so, when levels of pregnenolone decline, so too will the levels of the other hormones that are produced from it. For women, the majority of this decline happens with the onset of menopause – it is during these years, and the years beyond this change, that women begin to suffer from a host of different health issues and symptoms linked to a pregnenolone deficiency.

As well as being manufactured in the adrenal glands, pregnenolone is also produced in the cells of the liver, skin, ovaries and brain. However, pregnenolone levels in the brain are much higher than they are in the peripheral tissues. This is because, although much of the pregnenolone produced in the body is converted into other sex hormones, a certain amount of it remains unchanged, producing significant health benefits. And, in fact, a study published in the *Journal of Steroid Biochemistry and Molecular Biology* demonstrated that pregnenolone accumulates in the brain independently of sources in other areas of the body. If you recall, pregnenolone is derived from cholesterol. This 'top-of-the-range' hormone goes on to produce a cascade of hormones that includes DHEA (dehydroepiandrosterone), progesterone, testosterone and estrogens, aldosterone, and cortisol.

Pregnenolone is not only a precursor to all the other steroid hormones, it also belongs to a group called neurosteroids, as do DHEA and progesterone. Neurosteroids are important for regulating the balance between excitation and inhibition of neurons in the nervous system. To better understand, neurons communicate; they shoot out messages both through chemicals and electricity. These messages and impulses travel along the nervous system at breakneck speed. Neurons are responsible for daily functions that enable us to live: movement, moving the arm up and down, walking in the park, closing the fridge door, etc. Being able to respond to stimuli on time and react to impulses promptly is particularly important in life but being able to control this excitability is just as important. The regulation between these two functions, excitability and inhibition, is vital for the correct functioning of the brain and, therefore, the body. We need both; our messaging system needs 'sparks' but it also needs a 'brake' mechanism. Low levels of pregnenolone have been associated with dementia in elderly patients. Alzheimer's disease is the most common form of dementia.

In chapter 6 we spoke about statins and their association with brain dysfunction and cognitive impairment – again, if we take a look at the biochemical pathway and how statins totally disrupt this pathway, one could only logically predict that problems will occur. Going back on ourselves and doing some logical thinking here, statins lower cholesterol, pregnenolone is a derivative of cholesterol; pregnenolone is a precursor to a cascade of steroid hormones and is a neurosteroid; so, if we lower cholesterol, we will lower pregnenolone and, as a consequence, the production of all the other hormones will be decreased. Pregnenolone is a potent antioxidant and is neuroprotective. It is a neurosteroid. So, if this 'top-of-the-range' hormone and neurosteroid is lowered, we will take away its neuroprotective qualities. Put this together with the fact that hormones decline with age, and the brain situation doesn't look so good. Pregnenolone functions as a neuroprotective agent, guarding against cognitive impairment and Alzheimer's. Pregnenolone not only helps us cope with stress, it enhances concentration, improves memory and is a key player in mood control.

Pregnenolone is an androgen, as are DHEA and testosterone, and helps maintain and optimize muscle function. What are our muscles and brain going to do when there are inadequate levels of pregnenolone? Problems will occur.

A decrease in pregnenolone also causes symptoms such as feeling tired, being unable to cope with stress and having a lack of energy and enthusiasm. Other signs of below-optimal levels include low blood pressure, joint pains, frequent urination, cravings for salty foods, a loss of underarm and pubic hair, and increased risk of infections.

Apart from aging, the other known causes of a pregnenolone deficiency are low cholesterol levels (keep in mind that cholesterol-lowering drugs' function is to lower cholesterol) and hypothyroidism (this is when there are not enough thyroid hormones being secreted from the thyroid gland). If you recall, the body and its systems are dependent on the correct functioning of the thyroid gland, and nearly every organ in the body is profoundly affected by this important gland. When this 'communication mechanism' dysfunctions, pregnenolone production will also be affected. Remember, hormones talk to one another and are all interrelated, working in harmony for the sake of the body to maintain balance and, therefore, correct function. Another cause of low pregnenolone is a pituitary tumor; pregnenolone will make more cortisol and less of the other hormones to help the body deal with stress – remember the 'stealing process' we talked about in chapter 5 known as the pregnenolone-steal phenomenon?

Another important point to keep in mind is that when pregnenolone levels are low, the production of all the other steroid hormones will be decreased, provoking an imbalance. As a result, cholesterol production increases to try and correct the hormonal deficit (cholesterol produces hormones). Of course, when CLDs are involved, this process cannot happen – cholesterol cannot increase so hormones cannot be made in adequate quantities. The body needs these hormones like it needs cholesterol to function at optimum efficiency. The body is screaming out; it is desperately trying to correct this dysfunction (a decline in hormone production). The increased cholesterol production is a self-survival mechanism. Cholesterol (point of hormonal production) increases in an effort to produce more hormones. The whole body is interconnected: every system, organ, cell, mechanism and 'messaging machine' work together to form a network of harmony and perfect balance within the body. When this networking system is interrupted, the body cannot possibly maintain balance. This is when we see the onset of health issues appear.

The Major Functions of Pregnenolone in the Body

- Enhances nerve transmission and memory
- Assists in the repair of nerve damage
- Improves energy levels, both physically and mentally
- Improves sleep
- Regulates learning and memory, alertness and pain control

(modulates NMDA receptors)
- Increases resistance to stress
- Promotes mood elevation
- Reduces inflammation and pain
- Regulates balance between excitation and inhibition in the nervous system
- Modulates the neurotransmitter GABA (gamma-aminobutyric acid) – GABA is a part of the brain system which allows us to manage our moods, thoughts and actions and is critical to how we think and act. GABA calms and relaxes the brain, inhibiting excessive activity; it is the braking system we spoke about earlier.

It is no wonder, then, that taking a statin will inhibit all these bodily functions, causing the myriad of brain and muscle issues we see associated with this drug today.

Supplementing with bioidentical pregnenolone, on the other hand, when there is a deficiency, helps stimulate concentration and clarify thinking, prevents memory loss, fights depression, relieves arthritis and speeds healing. Pregnenolone supplementation is also used for, and has been seen to improve, autoimmune diseases such as rheumatoid arthritis, ankylosing spondylitis and lupus. Interestingly, when pregnenolone is used alongside other hormones such as estrogens, progesterone, testosterone or DHEA, a lesser dose of these hormones can be used as it is less physiologically disturbing.

DHEA (Dehydroepiandrosterone)

Pregnenolone goes on to create DHEA, which lies at the heart of the steroid family, and progesterone, by way of two separate pathways. By one pathway, pregnenolone leads to DHEA, which is then converted into testosterone, which then leads to the three primary estrogens: estradiol, estrone and, ultimately, estriol. In the other pathway, pregnenolone leads to another famous sex hormone, progesterone, which continues to produce a whole other family of non-sex steroid hormones known as glucocorticoids (including cortisol and cortisone). Whatever, all these steroid hormones need adequate cholesterol levels to be able to produce adequate amounts of hormones, which in turn maintain our health. It goes without saying that, if the production plants (cholesterol) are unable to produce enough products (hormones), either because of an age-related decline or because they have deliberately been inhibited with a statin drug, parts of the body will slowly but surely shut down and bankruptcy will occur.

DHEA is at its highest, optimal level at about aged twenty-five and is more than ten times higher than any other hormone in the body. Men produce higher levels of DHEA than women, largely because a significant amount is produced in the testes as well as the adrenal. However, their age-related decline of DHEA is more drastic than women's and, by the age of seventy, men have roughly equal amounts of DHEA to that of women. Importantly, optimal levels of DHEA protect both males and females from cardiovascular disease, although the hormone testosterone is more protective.

Women produce approximately 30% less than men, which may be why women seem to be more affected by adrenal stress than men. Women's ovaries contribute to a small amount of DHEA production, along with the brain and skin, but it is mostly the adrenal gland that is responsible for production.

One important benefit of DHEA, among many others, is that it stabilizes the negative effects of excess cortisol. If you recall, we mentioned previously (chapter 5) that there was a special relationship between DHEA and cortisol (stress hormone) known as the cortisol-to-DHEA ratio. Both these hormones are produced by the adrenal glands and are chiefly in charge of regulating the body's short-term stress response. DHEA has a complementary yet opposite relationship with cortisol: DHEA has a building effect (anabolic), whereas cortisol has a tearing-down (catabolic) effect on the body – both of these effects are essential to a well-functioning body.

The levels and ratios of both these hormones must be in balance to counteract one another and to enable you to obtain and maintain optimal health. When the ratios between these two hormones are out long-term, both mental and physical health issues will occur. We need optimal hormonal balance, not only between these two hormones but throughout the body, if we want to remain healthy.

There are various things that can contribute to DHEA deficiency

– here are a few: aging (menopause and andropause), cholesterol-lowering drugs, along with stress and smoking. Nicotine inhibits the production of a certain enzyme (11-beta-hydroxylase) needed to make DHEA; nicotine and cotinine also competitively inhibit multiple steps in testosterone biosynthesis (production).

An age-related decrease in DHEA can go on to decrease the production of all androgens by 50%. Individuals aged fifty to sixty have been seen to decrease serum DHEA by 70%-74% from its peak values registered in twenty- to thirty-year-old men and women, respectively. Age-related decline in DHEA has been linked to atrophy of the zona reticularis in the adrenal cortex (see diagram in chapter 5). The decreased function of the adrenals will, of course, interfere with DHEA production, which in turn will affect the production of the other hormones. Remember, hormones talk to one another, networking to achieve optimal health. When one hormone is out of synch, all the other hormones will also be out of synch. There will be a dysfunction within the network and, therefore, the body.

DHEA is a major marker for age and health, as well as the most prevalent steroid hormone in the human body and one of the most essential hormones in human health. In fact, with few exceptions, low or deficient DHEA is found in every illness including cancer, diabetes, depression, coronary artery disease, obesity, Alzheimer's and osteoporosis. Moreover, low DHEA-S concentration is independently and inversely related to death from any cause and, in particular, death from cardiovascular disease in men over fifty. Low levels of DHEA have also been linked to prostate disease, either benign prostatic hypertrophy (BPH) or prostate cancer. Remember, CLDs inhibit cholesterol production which, in turn, lowers DHEA production. However, please also remember that hormone production in general decreases with age. Hormonal balance is paramount to optimal health, in slowing the aging process and avoiding chronic disease.

DHEA, as stated previously, is a neurosteroid. It is also an androgen hormone (a group of hormones known as 'male' hormones even though women have these too). Being an androgen hormone, it helps stimulate muscle tissue and helps keep the muscle strong. It is well-known that statins adversely affect the muscles of the body – remember, the heart is a muscle.

The Major Functions of DHEA in the Body

- Assists in normalizing cholesterol levels
- Lowers triglycerides
- Helps you to better deal with stress
- Decreases allergic reactions
- Helps the body repair itself and maintain tissue
- Heightens lean body mass
- Heightens sense of well-being and energy
- Reduces insulin resistance – studies showed that, when supplementing with DHEA, there was a 30% decrease in insulin levels when compared to taking the diabetes drug Metformin alone
- Reduces spikes in blood sugar
- Supports and activates the immune system
- Increases brain function – helps reduce depression and enhances cognition
- Increases bone growth
- Decreases the formation of fatty deposits
- Helps with weight loss – lower obesity/waist-to-hip ratio
- Helps prevent blood clots
- Slows the progression of atherosclerosis
- Enhances libido and erectile ability.

It goes without saying that low levels of DHEA will cause a host of health issues, serious or otherwise. As you can see, there is a multitude of reasons why supplementing with DHEA is a good idea and taking a statin drug is not!

Note: DHEA is secreted into the bloodstream, like all steroid hormones, and is converted in the liver to DHEA-sulphate (DHEA-S). DHEA-S is a metabolite of DHEA and can be converted back into DHEA. DHEA-S is a far more accurate gauge in clinical testing as much more of it can be found in the blood. This in turn provides a more accurate gauge as to how much DHEA there is in the body.

Progesterone (Natural) Versus Progestins (Synthetic)

Progesterone is the oldest steroid hormone in the human body and is approximately 500 million years old on an evolutionary scale. All vertebrates have progesterone, although only in higher vertebrates is this hormone influential in assisting the reproductive cycle. Progestins, as stated at the beginning of chapter 7, are of the synthetic form (for example, medroxyprogesterone [Provera]) and they only became widely used in the mid-1970s together with Premarin (synthetic estrogen) as a combo drug known as PremPro.

Premarin came onto the market the same year it was approved by the FDA in 1942 but only became widely marketed in the 1960s and was designed to help menopausal symptoms. This horse-estrogen hormone was then found to cause cancer of the uterus (endometrial cancer) in epidemic proportions. Between 1970 and 1975, it was estimated that 15,000 women contracted endometrial cancer.

Instead of pulling this cancer-causing drug from their shelves, the pharmaceutical company decided to make another drug. They took the natural progesterone, converted it into progestin by chemically altering it so it could be patented, and called it medroxyprogesterone (Provera). These two drugs, Provera and Premarin, were then put together to prevent the equine estrogen causing uterine cancer and to increase the market share to women with uteruses. Thus, PremPro was born: Prem from Premarin and Pro from Provera.

However, this synthetic combo drug also proved fatal to women, increasing their risk of breast cancer and heart disease. PremPro was prescribed to menopausal women, in major part, to help with hot flashes, improve mood and sexual satisfaction, and help with the more long-term issues of cardiovascular disease, strokes and cognitive loss, which become more apparent post menopause. Although this combo drug did help to reduce hot flashes, it **did not**, however, achieve any of the other supposed benefits. The risks of taking this drug definitely outweighed the benefits, as was clearly demonstrated by the devastating WHI report (Women's Health Initiative Study) in 2002.

Again, progestins (synthetic progesterone) resemble the natural progesterone that is found in the body but, unlike bioidentical progesterone, they are not an exact copy of the human hormone. Progestins have been chemically altered in order to be patented. Provera and other progestins have a long list of negative side effects:

malignant breast tumors, loss of vision, thrombophlebitis, pulmonary emboli, cerebral thrombosis or stroke, increased birth defects, liver dysfunction or disease, excessive vaginal bleeding, epilepsy, migraine, asthma, heart and kidney failure, depression, aggravation of diabetes, acne, insomnia, fatigue, loss of libido, impaired thyroid function; the list goes on and on. The body has natural receptors (remember the lock-and-key setup) specifically for natural progesterone; there are no receptor sites in the body that are specifically for progestins, therefore these act as a foreign substance in the body and cause adverse side effects. Progestins do not reproduce the actions of natural progesterone; in fact, they interfere with the body's own production of progesterone and, once in the body, they can attach to many receptors sites, not just those for progesterone.

The most striking aspect of progestins (there are at least seven different types of progestins on the marketplace) is that they are not found in nature, neither in animal life nor plant life. Each of these synthetic molecules represents a metabolic endpoint, meaning that it is the 'end of the line' – there isn't, and can never be, a conversion point. They are foreign molecules that cannot be converted into cortisol, testosterone or estrogens. They cannot enhance the functionality of the body, only impede it – there are no advantages for us, only for the pharmaceutical companies. One word: money!

Progesterone – The True Hormone

Progesterone has been labeled as a 'female sex hormone', which is actually quite inappropriate. While it is true that females produce a greater amount than males, males also produce progesterone, albeit at lower concentrations. Progesterone per se, unlike estrogens and testosterone (we will discuss these two hormones in more detail later), do not dictate sex characteristics as they cause neither feminization nor masculinization definition. Progesterone has many direct and indirect roles in the body but its most basic role is to act as a precursor of cortisol, testosterone and estrogens. Natural progesterone, unlike progestins, has a metabolic endpoint, meaning that natural hormones can go on to be converted into the appropriate follow-on hormones and be metabolized, used and excreted efficiently by the body, causing no toxic build-up.

In short, just like cholesterol and pregnenolone, natural progesterone is a vital and essential factor for producing a homeostatic or balanced environment in the body. When the supply or production of progesterone slows because of, let's say, an age-related decline or interference by a cholesterol-lowering drug, all the steroid hormones and, more directly, the families of cortisol, estrogens and testosterone will be affected and this in turn will cause an imbalance.

Progesterone is fat soluble as it is made out of cholesterol, traveling through the blood as do all hormones. Once it reaches the cell membrane, it passes through it and, if there is a progesterone receptor, the appropriate cells will start to use the progesterone for various life-sustaining functions and processes. Unlike progestins, progesterone enhances the functionality of the body – there are enormous advantages to following nature.

Women produce progesterone in the ovaries and large amounts are produced in the luteal phase of the menstrual cycle. Progesterone also protects mother and baby during pregnancy. Men, on the other hand, produce very small amounts from the testicles. And, in males, progesterone remains stable to an extent (no monthly fluctuations) and is actually a part of the creation process of fully functional sperm. In both men and women, small amounts are produced in the adrenal glands where, again, it acts as a precursor to adrenal estrogens, testosterone and cortical steroids.

Both men and women need adequate amounts of progesterone. Progesterone is a natural diuretic and antidepressant, and has calming effects on the central nervous system. Progesterone production is closely linked to GABA, a neurotransmitter (remember, neurotransmitters, like neuropeptides, act as chemical messengers of information between nerve cells) which has a calming effect on the brain. Once progesterone has been metabolized, it binds to GABA receptors in the brain. For this reason, when progesterone levels are low, it may increase feelings of anxiety, irritability and anger. Neurotransmitters are extremely important for the production of sex hormones, including pregnenolone. Without the correct production and balance of specific neurotransmitters, there cannot be the correct production and balanced level of the sex hormones. The human infrastructure has been built so efficiently that all systems in the body are tightly interconnected – all systems work together, in harmony. When there is an age-related decline or when you inhibit, block or interfere with any system, then another system in the body will be affected. This system is part of the 'human network of health'. When progesterone levels are low, bioidentical progesterone can help support this downward process by suppressing mood swings and promoting total-body calmness. Progesterone can also act as a natural Prozac (popular antidepressant) for women.

Progesterone, along with estrogens, plays an important role in brain function and has been seen to be protective against Parkinson's disease. Like cortisol and DHEA, these two hormones, progesterone and estrogens, need to stay within a specific ratio. This ratio is not only vital to the menstrual cycle and fertility but also to overall mental and physical health and well-being.

Progesterone boosts mental acuity, cognitive performance and all mental function. It is neuroprotective and evidence suggests that progesterone may be a factor in the clinical treatment of traumatic brain injury. Supplementation shortly after injury to the brain and central nervous system (CNS) has been shown to significantly limit CNS damage, reduce loss of neuronal tissue and improve functional recovery. This evidence reinforces the fact that progesterone is protective against neurodegenerative diseases, the mechanism being the same. Again, disturb the cholesterol pathway with a CLD and we will lower progesterone and, thus, its neuroprotective qualities.

Progesterone assists thyroid function, helping to convert the inactive form (T4) to the active form (T3). The T4 hormone is less physiologically active and has to be converted into T3, the active hormone, in the body. If you recall, thyroid function affects nearly every organ in the body; when there is a dysfunction, the body and its system will dysfunction alongside.

Progesterone is also very helpful for the treatment of PMS and menopausal symptoms; it has anticancer properties, can help normalize and maintain correct blood-sugar levels, and protects the thymus gland which is a key gland for the immune system. It relaxes smooth muscle in the gut so foods can be broken down into nutrients that are then absorbed and used elsewhere in the body.

Progesterone is on the downstream pathway from cholesterol (below pregnenolone and alongside DHEA), therefore inhibiting cholesterol production will obviously provoke a negative impact on progesterone production. Statin drugs disrupt the production of cholesterol; all cholesterol drugs, including the older fibrates and newer statins, have been linked to increased rates of cancer. And, in fact, cancer of the breast has been seen to increase by 83%-143% in women taking statin drugs. In men, statin users were found to have as much as an 86% increased risk of developing prostate cancer than men who never took a statin drug, and the longer they took it, the higher their risk.

Progesterone in Men

Interestingly, progesterone levels in adult males are much higher throughout life than they are in postmenopausal women. However, up to now, little research has been done on progesterone in men.

As indicated earlier, progesterone is involved in the creation of fully functional sperm, being one of the regulatory mechanisms in its production. Progesterone-binding sites are found on the surface of sperm and, interestingly, defects in progesterone receptors in the sperm are found in infertile men. Progesterone is responsible for regulating calcium uptake in human sperm which, of course, should not come as a surprise considering it plays such a vital role in calcium metabolism and bone health, helping to avoid osteoporosis in both men and women. Importantly, progesterone inhibits the conversion of testosterone into dihydrotestosterone – dihydrotestosterone is the key player in prostate enlargement and cancer.

Major Functions of Progesterone in the Body

- Assists in normalizing cholesterol levels
- Has positive effect on sleep patterns
- Has a calming effect, helping to prevent anxiety, irritability and mood swings
- Helps build and form bone
- Helps with bladder function
- Balances the antagonistic effects of estrogens.

Estrogens

The Fear of the Unknown: Synthetic Versus Bioidentical

Once again, estrogens have been labeled a female hormone and are perhaps the more famous but certainly the more feared of the two female sex hormones. This would be due to the non-clarification or non-distinction between synthetic and bioidentical hormones. Over the last forty years or so, these synthetic hormones have been promoted as one and the same – they are not! And, over the last forty years or so, PremPro has generated huge sums of money for Wyeth Pharmaceuticals (in fact, billions of dollars; remaining at the top of the drug charts) when there is absolutely no clear evidence that they are safe and efficient.

As we mentioned previously, synthetic estrogens are concocted from the urine of pregnant mares and, although human hormones do contain some of the hormones found in pregnant mares' hormones (such as estradiol and estrone), they occur in extremely different proportions and certainly do not belong in the human body in these proportions.

Equine hormones – including estrone, equilin (the main horse estrogen which is secreted, along with eight other estrogens, only when the mare becomes pregnant and which, importantly, is never found in human estrogens at all) and its metabolites – are extremely potent. Women's bodies are not used to dealing with such powerful estrogens, especially in such large quantities. For one thing, the body cannot read them as it reads its own, they confuse the human infrastructure and total upset ensues. Therefore, it should come as no surprise that the ingestion of these estrogens in the body induces a hormonal imbalance and creates a dangerous scenario.

However, these alien estrogens are still estrogens – of a sort – and, as such, can do many things in the human body that estrogens are supposed to do, such as suppressing hot flashes and/or night sweats, as well as the progression of osteoporosis. However, due to their high potency, and along with their differences, they can cause great harm (beginning with fluid retention and tender breasts), going on to cause potentially fatal blood clots and cancers in the breast and uterus, all of which can be linked to excessive estrogenic activity. Put into plain English, Premarin has tissue-building estrogenic activity that is far more potent and longer lasting than natural endogenous or bioidentical estrogens. It is, therefore, extremely likely that these estrogenic overreactions, caused by Premarin, will promote tumor growth in the breast and uterus.

Bioidentical estrogens, when balanced and within the correct ratio with progesterone, do not cause such problems; they are natural and, therefore, understood, metabolized, used and excreted appropriately, in exactly the same way as endogenous estrogens are – they work in the same manner. They are safe and efficient and 'fit' the lock-and-key setup.

A Female or a Male Hormone?

Although classed as a female hormone, men have estrogens too, albeit at different concentrations. Men make estrogens out of testosterone (as do women), assisted by an enzyme called aromatase. Both men and women need estrogens in the body for correct functioning, good health and a feeling of overall well-being. Women need higher levels of estrogens but lower levels of testosterone, whereas men need lower levels of estrogens but higher levels of testosterone. Men require estrogens in large part because they help the brain function correctly. However, elevated levels of estrogens can be dangerous as they increase the risk of prostate cancer, stroke and heart disease. In women, the ratio is the other way around: when testosterone outweighs estrogens, it becomes toxic to the heart, increasing the risk of heart disease.

Estrogens: The True Hormone

Contrary to popular belief, estrogens are not a single hormone but are made up of a group of many different yet similar estrogens. The three main estrogens are: estrone (E1), estradiol (E2) and estriol (E3). However, they are far from being the only ones. Interestingly, estradiol and estrone can be converted into at least forty metabolic products.

Although the three forms of estrogen work together, each estrogen has its own varying activity; this is why all three have different names. Estradiol (E2) is the most potent form of estrogen and particularly 'feminizes' the body, being responsible for secondary sexual development (e.g. breasts and hips); it is twelve times more potent than estrone (E1) and eighty times stronger than estriol (E3).

Estradiol is converted from testosterone, which can then be converted into estrone and then back again into estradiol, something like a two-way street, to be converted when needed. Estriol is a by-product of both estrone and estradiol metabolism and cannot be converted; it is a one-way street and an 'end-of-the-line' product.

Although estriol is a very-low-potency or 'gentle' estrogen, research demonstrates that it may provide a natural, inbuilt and invaluable protection against the more potent cancer-causing estrogens (estrone and estradiol). High levels of both E1 and E2 have been associated with an increased risk of developing breast and uterine cancer as they stimulate these tissues. As mentioned previously, horse or equine hormones contain both E1 and E2 in vastly different proportions to human ones – of course, this is okay for the horse. What is also very interesting is that equine estrogens do not contain any estriol at all. Horses are nothing like us!

So, going back to humans, are we suggesting that there are good and bad estrogens? Not quite. There are, however, levels and ratios of hormones that must be adhered to which need to remain balanced and within optimal ranges to enable them to protect women and men, for that matter. When bodily systems perform optimally, the body takes care of itself; it has an 'inbuilt safeguard' to prevent the breakdown of these natural and vital protection mechanisms; it only needs the raw material to enable it to sustain itself. Understanding these bodily mechanisms is important to how you view your future health.

An important point to keep in mind when considering estrogen-sensitive cancers such as breast cancer is that there are alpha and beta receptors, otherwise known as ER-alpha and ER-beta. If you recall, receptor sites are places where hormones can bind or 'lock' onto. Estrone and estradiol mainly bind to alpha receptors (ER-alpha), which promotes cell proliferation and which can, in fact, lead to breast cancer. However, estriol mainly binds to beta receptors (ER-beta), which has the opposite effect, inhibiting breast-cell proliferation and preventing breast cancer. Cell proliferation is a natural process that has to occur in the body to enable us to survive; it is not a function that is there to deliberately cause cancer. When the correct amounts of estrogens, together with progesterone and its anticancer properties, are balanced, it creates a healthy environment, where cells can be created and proliferate in a healthy manner. When something goes wrong in this process and the 'fightback system' is weakened, problems can occur. One of these problems is the creation of a rogue cell that then takes on a life of its own instead of fitting into our normal structure. If that cell then replicates over and over again, its only purpose being to survive, we will have what is known as cancer. There has to be an even and correct balance of this process and, indeed, all processes within the body, to enable it to function and consistently protect itself efficiently.

Estrogens don't only sculpt the female body, they play an important role in many other processes. In fact, estrogens have over 400 crucial functions, and receptor sites can be found in the brain, muscle, bones, bladder, gut, uterus, vagina, breasts, eyes, heart, lungs and blood vessels. Estrogens assist in regulating body temperature and blood pressure, increasing sex drive, improving mood and preventing muscle damage.

Primarily, of course, estrogens are known to be responsible for the process of ovulation (releasing the ova from the ovaries), the role of the menstrual cycle and the transition into menopause. The correct balance of estrogens and progesterone leads to a normal monthly cycle with approximately twenty-eight days in between menstruations, which last roughly three to five days. When estrogens are predominant (something known as 'estrogen dominance'), this can lead to shorter intervals between menstruations as well as longer menstruation. Also, an overflow of estrogens compared to progesterone can provoke cancers such as uterine and breast cancer – it is a dangerous scenario. If progesterone is dominant, then we see the opposite: the interval between menstruations becomes longer and menstruation becomes short or may not happen at all. However, when we talk about either estrogen or progesterone dominance, it doesn't necessarily mean that either value is high (remember, all hormones decline with age) but, instead, the relative amount of either hormone is higher than the other – the ratio is off-balance.

Estrogens and progesterone work in tandem to regulate the body's release of insulin. E2 increases insulin sensitivity and improves glucose tolerance, whereas progesterone decreases insulin sensitivity and can cause insulin resistance. Women who have diabetes, in particular, need to make sure that their progesterone-to-estrogen ratio is normal. If you recall, statins can adversely affect insulin secretion and sensitivity, and can increase the risk of adult-onset type 2 diabetes by 10%-12%, with the risk being directly linked to the dose of the medication. Interfere with cholesterol production in any way and you interfere with hormone production, which will provoke an imbalance between these said ratios and other hormones. Inhibit cholesterol production by way of a cholesterol-lowering drug and you will get a downward cascade of bodily systems, which will bring with it a host of health issues, including diabetes.

Bone Health

Most of us know that bones serve as a reservoir for minerals – especially calcium – that may be needed by other parts of the body. However, it seems that most conventional doctors either prescribe bisphosphonates (such as Fosamax) that don't actually work, have some terrible side effects (see chapter 5) including heart issues, and cause a toxic build-up in the body, or they advise to take extremely large dosages of calcium, which is not very clever. Remember our discussion from chapter 1: calcium should always be taken alongside vitamin D3 and magnesium for heart health.

Yes, bones do need calcium for bone strength but the process is not as simple as that. Calcium cannot form new bone tissue all on its own; it needs a little help to complete the process – this includes help from the major sex hormones, estrogens, progesterone, testosterone, DHEA, and many others. In menopause, both estrogens and progesterone decline rapidly, although progesterone declines more drastically. Postmenopause, as levels continue to decline, elderly women find themselves at a higher risk than men. Women are affected eight times more than men by osteoporosis and their odds are one in three of each woman getting osteoporosis. In men, osteoporosis is due to a testosterone deficiency rather than a decline in estrogens. However, too little estrogens can also predispose a man to osteoporosis and bone fracture. Remember, estradiol is converted from testosterone – when testosterone levels are low, so will the level of estradiol; the effect is all in the correct balance for both men and women. It takes longer for osteoporosis to show up in men because of their bone structure (thicker and denser), needing more time to lose bone tissue before their bones become fragile. Men, however, are at a greater risk of remaining permanently disabled or dead if they break a hip. And, believe it or not, a man in his lifetime is more likely to suffer from a fracture related to osteoporosis than prostate cancer. Remember, the breakdown (osteoclast) and build-up (osteoblast) of bone is essential to bone health. With age, this process slows and begins to dysfunction in both sexes.

Healthy Lungs

One little-known benefit of estrogens is that they protect against the loss of lung surface area. Estrogens help protect against the loss and damage of alveoli (gas-exchange area of the lungs) which naturally occur with age. As women reach menopause, the loss of lung surface area accelerates; hormone restorative therapy can actually reverse this loss, maximize the lung's ability to absorb oxygen and rid itself of carbon dioxide. This is particularly important for athletic and non-smoking women who develop emphysema. It will, of course, also help women in their daily routine and movement, such as walking up and down stairs, doing the gardening, etc. Additionally, it helps keep the speaking and singing voice from 'aging' as quickly.

Pulmonary Hypertension (PH) in Women

Pulmonary hypertension (PH) is considered a serious health condition and occurs when the arteries that carry the blood to the lungs are constricted, disrupting and reducing blood flow. When the blood travels through the lungs, it collects oxygen so it can be delivered to all the organs, muscles and tissues in the body. When the arteries between the heart and lungs become narrow or the flow is constricted, the heart has to work twice as hard to pump the blood to the lungs. As time goes on, the heart weakens and blood circulation is diminished throughout the body. Pulmonary hypertension is life-threatening and can lead to heart failure and overall heart-health issues.

Overall, the incidence of pulmonary hypertension is higher in female patients, although they seem to have a better outcome, as shown by numerous animal studies. One study demonstrated that, after ovariectomy, the disease was exacerbated, suggesting that the female sex hormones played a significant protective role in this disease. However, and again, it is ER-alpha and ER-beta that are central to this protective role, albeit at a different stance to our previous discussion on breast cancer. What this means is that these two receptors have opposing effects in different tissues. E2 applies most of its biological effects through the two receptors (ER-alpha and ER-beta) which are abundantly expressed in the cardiopulmonary system. ER-beta has cardiopulmonary protective properties and vasodilatory properties in the heart and the lungs. On the other hand, ER-alpha, as stated previously, has pro-proliferative properties in certain tissues and cancers, whereas ER-beta exerts antiproliferative effects. The outcome is that both these subtype receptors are protective in their own way but they have to be balanced at the correct levels and function correctly to enable them to protect women from both cancer and PH.

Estrogens and the Brain

Estrogens are a group of powerful hormones that can affect the female brain enormously. And, in fact, there is not one brain cell that is not directly or indirectly sensitive to estrogens. Estrogens have neuroprotective functions, just like pregnenolone and the other steroid hormones. Estrogens are also known to help maintain memory in men when the ratios to testosterone are balanced (we will talk more about this ratio later). Again, they act as a neuroprotector, guarding a man's brain cells against damage and death.

One of their functions is to act as a natural antioxidant. Many studies have demonstrated that women with low levels of estradiol – the estrogen most responsible for maintaining brain function and which typically declines at menopause – develop brain issues. They may find that their retrieval time for facts, such as remembering someone's name, street address or telephone number, may not come to them as quickly as it once did and, in general, their memory may decline. Estrogens help maintain memory and cognitive function as well as increase the ability to learn new things. Furthermore, women on estrogens are half as likely to get Alzheimer's disease than women who are not on estrogens. Estrogens are a neuroactive hormone and react with receptors in the brain to modulate serotonin (a feel-good neurotransmitter) activity. Sudden and rapid changes in estrogen(s) levels can lead to decreased serotonin levels, which can provoke depression.

Skin Health

Beauty is directly related to a woman's hormonal levels. Hormones regulate all the organs, including the skin which is the largest organ of the body. As hormones decline, so does the quality, shine, plumpness, elasticity and texture of the skin. In particular, estrogens, along with progesterone, help preserve the skin's infrastructure. Declining estrogen(s) levels have been linked to a loss of collagen and elastin; this is why sagging, wrinkled and withered skin becomes part of the aging process.

Macular Degenerative Disease

Neurosteroids, such as pregnenolone, DHEA, corticosteroids and sex hormones, all play a role in visual function. However, estrogens in particular have been linked to age- and gender-associated ocular disease and the prevention of retinal injury. Low estrogen(s) levels are harmful to the retina and have been implicated in the development of macular degeneration in women who enter menopause at an early age. Drugs such as tamoxifen, an anti-cancer drug which blocks estrogens production, is harmful to the retina. Block estrogen(s) in whatever way, whether through a statin drug or an anti-cancer drug such as tamoxifen, and you will damage the retina.

The retina is considered as an external part of the brain. It has its own receptor sites and, like the brain, it is able to make its own hormones, many of which play a key role in it. Remember, to make hormones we need cholesterol. Cholesterol can be synthesized (manufactured) in the neural retina and then transformed into a cascade of hormones. This implicates that hormonal production and, therefore, cholesterol production, is intrinsically linked to macular degenerative disease and the health of the eye. And, in fact, hormones are part of the biophysiology of vision itself.

Macular degenerative disease is one of the many adverse effects that have been linked to the statin drug another reason why we should think twice about taking any cholesterol-lowering drug. Inhibit cholesterol and we lower hormone production along the way!

Note: Importantly, estradiol has been shown to lower blood pressure in postmenopausal women and, because of it, antioxidant powers. Estradiol inhibits oxidation of LDL, which is an initiating event in atherosclerosis.

Women who have inadequate amounts of estrogens have been seen to have a much larger area of stroke and to heal less quickly. If estrogen(s) levels are adequate or optimal, the area of damage is smaller and heals at a greater rate. Hormones keep the damaging effect of a stroke in check.

Adequate and balanced estrogen(s) levels have been seen to increase female life expectancy, protecting against an increased risk of overall mortality.

Causes of Estrogen(s) Deficiency

The primary cause of an estrogen(s) decline is age. This includes perimenopause, menopause, premature ovarian decline, andropause and, of course, cholesterol-lowering drugs. When hormone production is muted, they can no longer do their job and protect us as they should.

Major Functions of Estrogens in the Body

- Decrease fatigue
- Decrease platelet stickiness
- Assist in normalizing cholesterol levels
- Assist in maintaining memory
- Assist in maintaining potassium levels
- Assist in maintaining healthy bones
- Assist with the absorption of calcium, magnesium and zinc
- Improve sleep
- Increase endorphins
- Increase insulin sensitivity and improve glucose tolerance

- Increase growth hormone
- Increase serotonin levels
- Act as a potent antioxidant
- Control menopausal symptoms (hot flashes, insomnia, vaginal dryness)
- Assist gut health, maintaining a favorable environment for the growth of good bacteria (lactobacilli)
- Help restore correct pH of the vagina, which prevents urinary tract infections (UTIs)
- Increase GABA (a calming neurotransmitter)
- Increase manual speed and dexterity
- Increase blood flow
- Maintain the blood-brain barrier
- Act as a natural calcium blocker to help keep arteries open
- Dilate small arteries
- Enhance magnesium uptake and utilization
- Help maintain the elasticity of the arteries.

In summary, when estrogen(s) levels are low (either due to an age-related decline or because of a cholesterol-lowering drug), their neuroprotective and cardioprotective qualities will be decreased. There will also be an increased risk of cancers due to an imbalance and/or decline of hormones and a weakening of the immune system. If you recall, hormones are the most fundamental molecule in building a healthy, functional immune system.

Testosterone

Now we get to the so-called 'male' hormone, the almighty testosterone. Testosterone, like estrogens, dictates sex characteristics as it causes masculinization definition. Testosterone is the hormone that makes males men – bulky and muscular – and estrogens are a group of hormones that make females women – curvaceous and sexy. This is why men have higher levels of testosterone but lower estrogens than women, and vice versa, but it is by no means an 'all-over' male hormone as it plays many important functions in both sexes.

Testosterone, a major androgen, comes from the all-important hormone DHEA and two intermediate hormones, androstenediol and androstenedione, which in turn lead to the three primary estrogens mentioned earlier: E2, E1 and, ultimately, E3. Estradiol can be made from two direct pathways, some of which begins as testosterone, as mentioned previously, while the rest is converted from androstenedione and estrone. There is a continual chain of events happening in the endocrine system and, indeed, the whole body – every process has to fit together in the correct order and the right way. It is a highly complex assembly line; no engineer could ever have contemplated writing instructions for such an intricate and complex process.

In women, testosterone is manufactured in the adrenal glands and ovaries. As women age, the ovaries produce less testosterone and so are more dependent on the adrenals and the production of DHEA for their testosterone. In men, testosterone is manufactured in the testes and, to a lesser extent, the adrenals. Levels begin to drop steadily, by 1% per year, from the age of thirty and older. The major difference between hormonal decline in males and that in females is that men lose their testosterone at a slower rate and over a period of thirty years, whereas women lose both their sex hormones (estrogens and progesterone) at a much more dramatic rate and within a period of five years. This would account for the hyper-acute symptoms that women suffer during this transition, while men's symptoms are less notable. A man is aware that something is wrong but does not really understand the significance of this slow-and-steady decline.

In men, testosterone is needed for erection, ejaculation and fertility – a man is incapable of an erection when estrogens outweigh testosterone. Once again, there is a ratio that has to be adhered to: the testosterone-estrogens ratio in men and the estrogens-testosterone ratio in women. Women naturally have a high-estrogens-to-low-testosterone ratio and men naturally have a high-testosterone-to-low-estrogens ratio. When this ratio is out, in either men or women, they spiral into a decline. It is this ratio that keeps them looking good and feeling healthy. Almost every disease starts with a hormonal decline in both men and women. It's no wonder statins have so many adverse effects, deleterious or otherwise.

As an example, in men, when levels of testosterone are low, they are up to 51% more likely to develop frailty, a condition linked to early death, compared to those with higher levels. Declining testosterone levels have been associated with osteoporosis, reduced sexual functioning and performance, muscle atrophy and weakness, increased fat mass, metabolic syndrome, increased risk of diabetes, depression, cognitive impairment and an increased risk of developing Alzheimer's disease.

When testosterone and estrogens are optimized and balanced within the correct ratios, many age-related disorders can be avoided and sometimes reversed. These include cardiovascular disease, improved sex drive, bone density, strength, muscle mass, body composition, mood, cognition, red-blood-cell formation and an improved quality of life.

The major and most direct causes of a testosterone deficiency are the aging process (including menopause and andropause) and cholesterol-lowering drugs. Surgical menopause, chemotherapy, childbirth and birth-control pills also affect testosterone production.

Testosterone and Cardiovascular Health

Millions of dollars are spent on high-tech procedures such as bypass surgery and balloon angioplasty, neither of which truly address the problem. Both Dr Dzugan and I believe that the major component of heart disease is a hormonal imbalance, which in turn provokes a dysregulation between the catabolic (breakdown) and anabolic (repair) process (more on this later).

Unfortunately, the majority of doctors practicing today are unaware of the role testosterone and other hormones play in the maintenance of men's cardiovascular health (and women's, for that matter), believing that they are actually dangerous to the heart. This may be due to two separate misconceptions. The first is that elevated levels of testosterone (compared to estrogens) in women can be toxic for the heart which, of course, is true. However, in women, testosterone and estrogens per se are needed for overall heart health. We should be aware that both sexes react differently to testosterone and estrogens alike. Just as men react differently to estrogens, women react differently to testosterone – it is all to do with the ratios. The second reason is the misuse and overuse of anabolic steroid drugs by some athletes and bodybuilders, such as methyltestosterone, which have been associated with serious heart disease and have also been found to be carcinogenic. The use of natural testosterone taken in physiological amounts does not present such issues.

Truth be known, when it is given in physiological amounts and is natural, testosterone keeps the heart strong and pumping efficiently. It strengthens and protects the heart by nurturing the cardiac muscle which, by the way, has more testosterone receptor sites than any other muscle in the body.

As stated previously, elevated estrogens in men increase the risk of cardiovascular disease. Both low testosterone and high estradiol have been associated with cardiovascular disease. However, it is not necessarily the absolute values (levels) but the testosterone-to-estradiol ratio that is the issue here. As testosterone declines and the active amount (creating activity in all cells, brain, muscle, heart, bone, gonads, etc., accounting for approximately 2% or 3% of total testosterone) in a man's blood decreases, it gives way to a higher ratio or proportion of estradiol. By the time a man reaches sixty, he can have more estrogens than a fifty-year-old woman. This ever-increasing proportion of estrogens to testosterone increases blood-clotting factors and narrowing of the coronary arteries, increasing the risk of heart attack and stroke. (It is the opposite in women: higher testosterone-to-estrogens ratio.)

Restoring testosterone levels in aged men is important for protecting against mortality and heart-related events. A recent large population-based cohort study demonstrated that long-term testosterone replacement therapy was associated with a decreased risk (note, not increased risk) for cardiovascular disease, and the longer the treatment, the more protective it was against mortality and heart-related events.

Testosterone and the Brain

When testosterone levels are low in men, they are far more likely to suffer from brain issues such as Alzheimer's disease. And, in fact, the development of memory loss has been associated with age-related testosterone decline. Testosterone has even been seen to preserve and assist in new-brain-cell growth in the hippocampus – the part of the brain that processes memory and loses neurons with age. Various studies show that a decline in testosterone levels can affect different types of memory. These include visual and verbal memory, spatial and mathematical interpretation. Conversely, higher levels are linked to better memory and cognitive function, including those just mentioned.

Low testosterone levels lead to increased brain (neuron) cell damage and death, higher antibody levels and an increased production of the amyloid-B protein which has been linked to Alzheimer's and other forms of dementia. Interestingly, supplementation with testosterone has shown that the overall quality of life increases in patients suffering from Alzheimer's. Testosterone treatment has also been seen to help neurons improve from impaired function. Low levels of testosterone have also been associated with Parkinson's disease and amyotrophic lateral sclerosis, more commonly known as Lou Gehrig's disease.

Just as estrogens are a major protector of the brain in women, testosterone is a major protector of the brain in men. However and whatever, for testosterone and/or E2 (estradiol) to work well, they have to be balanced within the correct ratios, in both men and women. Both these hormones play a role in how well the body and brain work, or don't work. Testosterone is important to cognition, not only in men but also in women, as is estradiol – they are both neuroprotectors when balanced and within their correct ratios.

Testosterone and Cancer

Testosterone and prostate cancer is a 'hot topic' – who says high testosterone levels cause prostate cancer? It's a myth. High testosterone levels do not fuel cancer but low levels can. Here is a simple question: how come prostate cancer and the progressive growth of the prostate, which is a highly androgen-dependent organ, are more commonly seen in men as they age and reach andropause just as their testosterone levels are beginning to decline? Something is wrong. In fact, low testosterone levels actually increase the risk of prostate cancer and have been associated with a more aggressive prostate cancer. On the other hand, elevated levels of testosterone prior to the onset of prostate cancer have been seen to increase survival rate. And not only were higher levels of testosterone associated with less incidence of prostate cancer but also with a longer lifespan.

There is no clinical or scientific data that supports the concept that high testosterone levels increase the risk of either BPH (benign prostatic hyperplasia) or prostate cancer. When men's testosterone levels decline, they see a rise in PSA (prostate specific antigen) and along comes the increased risk of prostate cancer. PSA is a blood test that, when elevated, may indicate an enlarged prostate gland or cancer. A fairly recent study showed that, when testosterone levels were restored, it not only lowered PSA levels in middle-aged men and older but also reversed prostate growth. And a more recent, large population-based cohort study demonstrated that, when testosterone levels were restored, there was no increased risk over short-term exposure and the risk decreased with increasing exposure. And, in fact, with long-term exposure, prostate cancer decreased by 40%.

Testosterone and Erectile Dysfunction (ED)

When there is a testosterone imbalance, a man will be unable to get a good erection as the blood vessels in the pelvis will be unable to dilate to achieve the desired result – this is a good biomarker for testosterone deficiency. Another clear biomarker of inadequate testosterone is when there is no 'early-morning rise'. Erectile capacity is an indication of health and we are not just talking sexually. These reflex erections, which happen every so often all night long, are related to the sensitivity of vascular and neural tissues. Healthy heart, healthy mind, healthy man. Apart from being critical to sexual function, testosterone is also important to sexual fantasy that comes directly from the brain. When levels are low, a man may feel depressed and have very low libido with very little fantasy.

ED is an indicator that the brain and the heart are not dilating effectively. A man is then two to three times more likely to have a stroke or heart attack. Men with low testosterone will have more severe strokes, with much more damage, just as women with low or imbalanced estrogens will. Testosterone is a major vasodilator for the brain, heart and pelvic vasculature; these central critical arteries are extremely sensitive to hormone input.

In women, testosterone is needed for sex drive and strong libido, along with progesterone and estrogens. The female sex hormones, estrogens and progesterone, are significant in maintaining women's organs healthy and in good working order, keeping vaginal tissue thick, lubricated and free from infections, and helping them to enjoy pain-free intercourse. However, estrogens do not have any direct effect on libido, whereas testosterone and the other androgens (androstenedione, androstenediol, DHEA, DHEA-S) do, being mainly responsible for charging the batteries of sexual desire, and encouraging enjoyment, fantasy and orgasm. Testosterone also stimulates love and affection, as well as sexual emotions. Approximately 86% of women report a decrease in sexual interest with menopause.

Note: Supplementing with bioidentical testosterone is important for women who have had a hysterectomy, otherwise known as surgical menopause. Surgical menopause has a much more dramatic and immediate effect on the body than natural menopause as the body is suddenly thrown into a state of confusion. If you recall, testosterone is manufactured in the ovaries and adrenal glands. After a hysterectomy, the majority of women have extremely low testosterone levels.

Testosterone, Insulin Resistance and Diabetes

Testosterone is one of the major regulators of sugar, fat and protein metabolism in the body. When, in men, there is too much estrogen(s) compared to testosterone, it can provoke insulin resistance (just as an imbalance of estrogens to progesterone can in women), which can lead to diabetes type 2 as its (testosterone) 'antagonistic' properties to the stress hormones, cortisol and adrenalin, are weakened. Low testosterone levels can result in weight gain (in particular around the middle), high blood pressure, and increased cholesterol and triglycerides. Testosterone is of great benefit to men with diabetes and has also been found to be effective for complications related to this health issue, such as diabetic retinopathy, gangrene and peripheral vascular disease. Restoring testosterone levels can save a life and a limb.

If you recall, insulin resistance and diabetes are significant risk factors in heart disease. A hormonal imbalance and, in particular, a decline in testosterone are a greater independent risk factor for heart disease and stroke than a male's family history, total cholesterol or cigarette smoke.

Insulin resistance is also a major issue in degenerative diseases such as cancer and Alzheimer's disease.

An overload of estrogens can occur for a variety of reasons: increased aromatase with age (aromatase is an enzyme that converts testosterone to estrogens and is found in fat cells – so the more overweight a person is, the more estrogens he or she will produce); weight gain; a decreased function or effectiveness of the liver (which metabolizes estrogens) due to prescription drugs; and a deficiency of zinc which inhibits aromatase levels. Unfortunately, men can get caught up in a 'crossfire effect' where more estrogens are made by aromatase due to increased weight gain which is due to low testosterone levels. The end result is an ever-depleting testosterone level with an increased estradiol level, thus reaching unsafe ranges. Additionally, estrogens increase the production of a hormone known as sex-hormone-binding globulin (SHBG) which binds testosterone, causing less bioactive-testosterone availability, which in turn leads to a continual downward cycle. Just imagine how taking a statin drug would impact testosterone levels even further.

Major Functions of Testosterone in the Body

- Helps lower excess body fat
- Helps tone muscle, so skin is less saggy
- Helps increase muscle mass and strength
- Protects bone by decreasing bone deterioration
- Acts as an antidepressant as it elevates norepinephrine in the brain
- Helps maintain memory
- Increases self-confidence, a sense of emotional well-being and motivation
- Protects the heart and its function
- Boosts libido, sexual functioning and performance.

Cortisol

Cortisol, the stress hormone, lies on the progesterone pathway which produces a whole family of non-sex-steroid hormones known as glucocorticoids, including cortisol. It is produced in the adrenal glands

– the same gland that produces DHEA. Cortisol, thyroid, insulin and adrenaline are all essential to life; without them we could not survive for long. Estrogens, progesterone, testosterone, pregnenolone and DHEA, on the other hand, are responsible for fine-tuning and a feeling of well-being. Hormones communicate with each other and need to be in balance for us to feel well and for our bodies to work at optimum. Of course, aging and the money-making statins interfere with this communication network big time!

This life-essential hormone converts amino acids into glucose energy, enhances memory functions, lowers sensitivity to pain and has anti-inflammatory and immunosuppressive properties.

In today's world, stress is continual and relentless, there is no getting away from it – from pressures at work, organizing the family, rushed lunches, financial problems, to being stuck in traffic or just not having enough hours in the day. Stress upon stress! Stress activates the sympathetic nervous system which works alongside the parasympathetic nervous system to regulate many homeostatic mechanisms within the body. In other words, these two nervous systems work together to maintain balance within the body and its systems. The sympathetic nervous system is an energy-giver and is known as the 'fight-or-flight' system (activated under stress), whereas the parasympathetic system is a calming system that brings the body back into equilibrium or homeostasis after the stress situation has passed.

The sympathetic and parasympathetic nervous systems are directly connected to the hypothalamic-pituitary-adrenal (HPA) axis through a feedback loop mechanism. The HPA axis is key to achieving homeostasis; each component works in concert and is affected by environment and lifestyle. If we have been out of sync – such as in a hormonal imbalance, not sleeping well, poor diet or high stress levels – the HPA axis will be off-balance. When these systems are 'out', the body struggles enormously to function correctly and, in fact, finds it almost impossible. Add the aging process and a cholesterol-lowering drug to this 'stress equation', plus the imbalance of hormone levels it will create, and you've just topped the mountain and, of course… fallen off.

An important point to keep in mind is that cortisol levels fluctuate throughout the day and, of course, there is a good reason for this – the body always knows best. Cortisol output is normally highest in the morning then, throughout the day, it has a mid-value, while during the night the output drops off significantly. Of course, if a person works nightshifts or sleeps at different times of the day, this pattern may change. When we say 'cortisol output is normally highest in the morning' we don't mean high cortisol as in long-term cortisol dominance but as part of the daily cycle of cortisol or of a physiological function.

Interestingly, there is a huge misconception evolving around cortisol: most medical doctors, including the most prominent, believe that cortisol levels rise with age. However, there are many studies showing that cortisol production remains either stable or, if not, declines with age. One particular study, done in 2005, conducted by Life Extension Foundation and based on data of 246 men and women aged nineteen to ninety-three, showed that cortisol levels declined with age and that the majority of patients possessed less than optimal levels of cortisol. An optimal level was found in only 28.04% of patients and 17.88% had a cortisol level on the low side. On the other hand, only 7.72% actually had elevated cortisol levels.

In chapter 5 we discussed the devastating effects long-term and chronic stress can have on the body. Cortisol is an essential hormone for maintaining optimal health and an impaired secretion and regulation of this hormone can have devastating effects on the body. Chronically elevated levels of cortisol (cortisol dominance) can be dangerous but, just as importantly, low levels can be just as detrimental to our health as high levels.

Continual and long-term pouring of cortisol into the bloodstream is consequently highly destructive. It leads to impaired cognitive performance such as concentration, memory and problem-solving. Along comes thyroid suppression, which can cause blood-sugar imbalances and may lead to insulin resistance. We see elevated blood pressure as cortisol regulates blood pressure and cardiovascular function. We may also see a decrease in bone density and muscle tissue, together with an increase in abdominal fat, which is associated with various health risks including heart attack and stroke. Sleep problems may occur, along with fatigue, premature aging and, behaviorally, emotions such as depression, anxiety, irritability and sadness.

However, diminished cortisol levels offer some of these very same symptoms, including insomnia, fatigue and depression. Decreased cortisol levels have also been associated with behavioral disorder, aggression and increased stroke risk. And, even more frighteningly, low cortisol levels have been correlated to repeated suicide attempts, violent criminal behavior and psychopathic tendencies. Chemical sensitivities and allergies have also been linked to subpar adrenal stress index (this simply refers to the ratios between cortisol and DHEA that we discussed in chapter 5). As with the estrogens-to-progesterone ratio in women and the testosterone-to-estrogens ratio in men, neither low nor high levels are good – balance and optimization of each ratio is key to optimal health and the prevention of symptoms.

Cortisol and the Brain

Impaired cortisol secretion and regulation ages the brain. High levels of cortisol or cortisol dominance impairs cognitive function and can affect the way we think. It touches our memory function, our learning abilities and our creativity; we may have more difficulty in solving problems, our reaction time may be slower, we may become forgetful and have difficulty in making decisions, and we may have more difficulty in recalling and retrieving information. Our brain is one of the body parts most affected by stress: when cortisol levels are high, or we have cortisol dominance, our body produces more free radicals which damage neurons, affecting our ability to think and remember things. Additionally, cortisol dominance is correlated to a deterioration of the hippocampus, which is the part of the brain that processes memory. However, when eliminating or removing the source of stress, the hippocampus has been seen to be able to grow back. This, of course, is easier said than done; you need to make a concerted effort to have a more relaxed, less stressful lifestyle, together with restoring hormone levels and not taking CLDs. The body is under a continual and high stress load when there is a decline in hormone levels. Also, elevated cortisol levels may directly contribute to Alzheimer's disease.

Cortisol and the Insulin Connection

Cortisol works in tandem with insulin from the pancreas, making sure glucose gets to the cells where it can be burned for energy. Cortisol makes sure adequate levels of glucose are in the blood, while insulin, being the platinum key, unlocks the cell membranes to get glucose into the cells. Our body relies on glucose as the most consistent form of energy.

When there is abnormal adrenal function due to long-term or chronic stress, it may alter the ability of the cells to produce the energy we need for the activities of everyday living. If getting up in the morning is difficult or if energy levels are low during the day, it may be due to abnormal adrenal rhythms and poor blood-sugar regulation.

When there is stress-induced cortisol secretion, we get high cortisol levels to low DHEA levels. As we mentioned previously, cortisol dominance can be connected to increased central body fat and can create insulin resistance; long-term insulin resistance can cause diabetes type 2. If insulin resistance is left unchecked, it can lead to metabolic syndrome or Syndrome X. If this condition develops, the sugar that would normally be used for energy is stored as fat instead. This is when we start to see an increase in weight, especially around the abdomen – women getting thicker around the stomach, waist and thighs, and men becoming 'potbellied'. When DHEA is administered (or supplemented with), it has been seen to reduce the accumulation of central or abdominal visceral fat and protect against insulin resistance – insulin resistance increases the risk of heart disease. Remember, one cause of heart disease is having excess sugar floating about in the bloodstream. Also, statins increase diabetes and the longer you take them, the higher the risk (the JUPITER trial demonstrated an incredible 25% increased risk of new-onset diabetes). One side effect of this medication is that it increases blood-glucose levels (hyperglycemia). Statins impair pancreatic beta-cell function (where insulin is produced) and, therefore, decrease insulin sensitivity; continual insulin sensitivity will eventually provoke diabetes type 2.

Stress and Depression

Another example of subpar adrenal stress index is the association with depression. In an adult population, a high cortisol-to-DHEA ratio has been linked to unipolar depression and, in adolescents, a high cortisol-to-DHEA ratio was predictive of persistent major depression prior to the onset of unipolar depression. Also, a high morning cortisol-to-DHEA ratio in older men has been associated with negative mood, high anxiety and a less than optimal cognitive function. Also, depression and cognitive deficits, both of which characterize severe mood disorders, have been associated with elevated cortisol.

Cortisol Rhythms and Aging Skin

Our skin regenerates mainly during the night, so, if you want to achieve optimal skin health, it is essential to have normal cortisol rhythms. When there are higher night cortisol values, there is less skin regeneration. Cortisol-to-DHEA ratio needs to be balanced. Sleep is so important. Poor quality of sleep or deprivation affects the endocrine system and hormone production. If we don't sleep, our hormones get mixed up and, if there is a hormonal imbalance, we cannot sleep. Low morning cortisol and elevated evening cortisol have been associated with insomnia.

Cortisol and Blood Pressure

Correct cortisol regulation is important to maintaining blood pressure and cardiovascular function. Remember that high blood pressure damages the endothelium (the inner lining of the arteries) and it is the functional and structural integrity of the arteries that keeps us safe. When the endothelium is damaged or injured, and therefore compromised, it cannot function as it should. The words 'cortisol dominance' and 'heart attack' go hand in hand; chronically, high cortisol levels lead to hypertension and nearly always lead to heart disease, heart attack and stroke.

Major Functions of Cortisol in the Body

- Influences PTA (pituitary-thyroid-adrenal) system
- Balances blood sugar
- Controls weight
- Affects immune-system response

- Influences bone turnover rate
- Affects stress reaction
- Assists in protein synthesis
- Helps you sleep
- Influences DHEA/insulin ratio
- Influences estrogens and testosterone ratio
- Is an anti-inflammatory.

Thyroid-Adrenal Function and the Cholesterol Connection

Although the thyroid hormones T4 and T3 are not directly on the cholesterol pathway, they can, however, affect cholesterol synthesis. Thyroid affects every metabolic function in the body and, therefore, our overall health greatly.

As mentioned previously (see under 'Thyroid Gland' in this chapter), the thyroid gland releases the iodine-containing hormones thyroxine (T4) and triiodothyronine (T3), their major function being to influence the metabolism of cells – in other words, they help the cell machinery to produce energy. The thyroid gland produces much more T4 (approximately 80%) than T3 (approximately 20%), which has to be converted once inside the cells of the body. T3 is much more active than T4 (about 300% more active) and it is T3 that actually increases the metabolism inside the cells.

In chapter 5 we spoke about long-term stress causing adrenal exhaustion. When the adrenals are exhausted, the production of adrenal hormones is drastically reduced – pregnenolone, DHEA, progesterone, estrogens, testosterone and aldosterone (pregnenolone is a precursor to all these hormones) all decline in favor of cortisol. We named this phenomenon 'pregnenolone steal' (remember, pregnenolone is directly produced from cholesterol); this, in turn, will create a physiological demand for more cholesterol to be produced. When there is a decline in hormone production, we see an increase in cholesterol synthesis.

The thyroid gland is directly affected by the adrenal hormones, therefore thyroid problems may occur due to adrenal maladaptation, due to a damaged adrenal gland. The adrenals assist in the conversion of thyroid hormones to the active form (T3).

When there is an adrenal-maladaptation scenario, the thyroid hormone (T4) may become stored and therefore unavailable for the body to use. If T4 is unavailable, it cannot be converted into the active form T3. Decreased or low levels of T3 can cause an increase in cholesterol levels because low levels of T3 cause less cholesterol to be transported out of the blood.

If your thyroid isn't functioning adequately (hypothyroidism), it will affect the heart's ability to pump efficiently. Hypothyroidism, or low thyroid, can also lead to an enlarged heart and heart failure. It is sad that most cardiologists immediately pull out the prescription pad to prescribe statins, instead of taking a deeper look at the hormonal system along with the thyroid hormones.

Thyroid hormones specifically inhibit prolactin synthesis and decrease the levels of prolactin messenger ribonucleic acid (RNA) in cultured pituitary cells. Prolactin is a unique hormone released by the anterior part of the pituitary gland and serves as an informational hub for different catecholamines (dopamine, serotonin) and hormones (estrogens, progesterone, testosterone, thyroid, etc.). This information comes through positive and negative feedback. Thyroid hormones reduce the number of thyroid releasing hormone (TRH) receptors and inhibit prolactin messenger RNA synthesis. Any change in the function of thyroid hormones can affect steroid hormones that are involved in prolactin physiology and, of course, will also change cholesterol biosynthesis.

Correct thyroid function is indirectly linked to the tightly controlled cholesterol mechanism. We seem to forget that the body is a working, functioning network of systems that literally feeds or functions from and/or through the other. When one is messed up, the other will fail and fall into default. It is essential that all of the hormonal glands (thyroid, adrenals, ovaries, testes, hypothalamus and pituitary) are functioning at their respective optimal levels because they are so closely related and work in synergy. It is impossible to achieve optimum health until the entire hormonal system is functioning correctly. When a system, and therefore a process, in the body goes into default, it will automatically have a knock-off effect on some other part of the body by way of a feedback loop mechanism.

Whatever, it is vitally important to understand that good thyroid function is essential to hormonal balance, and that hormonal balance is essential to correct cholesterol synthesis. Age, stress and cholesterol-lowering drugs all affect hormonal balance and, therefore, synthesis.

Vitamin D3

We already spoke about vitamin D3 in chapter 1 and the fact that it is a hormone (produced in the body) rather than a vitamin (obtained through diet). However, vitamin D3 can be obtained through a few foods such as red meat and fish, but most of it is delivered by way of direct sunlight and, in fact, vitamin-D production begins in the skin rather than in the mouth. If you recall, the body is capable of manufacturing vitamin D3 simply through exposure to sunlight. If you are depending on sunlight, rather than diet or supplementation, to get your vitamin D, then the recommended amount is fifteen to twenty minutes a day, with 40% of the skin surface exposed. Vitamin-D deficiency is a global health problem and nearly a billion people worldwide are vitamin-D deficient or insufficient. This includes those living in warmer climates.

Vitamin D3 is essential to overall health. It is a secosteroid neurohormone and therefore has neurotransmitter and neurological functions. It functions like all steroids by turning genes on and off and, in fact, regulates the functions of over 200 genes; some of these genes regulate cancer-cell growth and differentiation, protecting us against cancers such as breast, colon, skin and prostate. These genes also regulate cell death and limit the growth of tumor blood supplies. Vitamin D3 has receptors throughout the body, including bones, pancreas, intestine, kidneys, brain, spinal cord, reproductive organs, thymus, adrenal glands, pituitary gland and the thyroid gland. This statement alone reinforces the fact that this vitamin is vital to overall health.

Vitamin D3 is a product of cholesterol, therefore if there is a deficiency of this hormone, it can affect cholesterol levels (cholesterol will increase to make up for vitamin D3 deficiency). Vitamin D3 synthesis declines greatly with age, mainly because the concentration of 7-dehydrocholesterol in the skin declines. And, of course, cholesterol-lowering drugs such as statins, or HMG-CoA reductase-inhibitors, which are designed to inhibit the synthesis of 7-dehydrocholesterol and cholesterol, will therefore affect the synthesis of vitamin D3.

Vitamin D3 plays a myriad of important roles in the body and is best known for its role in calcium metabolism and bone health. Vitamin D3 facilitates the absorption of calcium from the small intestine; if there is insufficient vitamin D3, calcium cannot be integrated into the bones. There has to be enough vitamin D3 for calcium to function correctly, otherwise the bones will become soft. Taking calcium without sufficient vitamin D3 (and, of course, magnesium – always take magnesium when taking calcium) may actually weaken the bones over time.

Deficient vitamin D3 levels have been linked to practically every health- and age-related disorder in the body, including diabetes, hypertension, depression, fibromyalgia, chronic-fatigue syndrome, osteoporosis, chronic inflammation and Alzheimer's. Recent research indicates that a deficiency plays a role in seventeen varieties of cancers, as well as heart disease, stroke, autoimmune diseases, birth defects and periodontal disease. Vitamin D3 is vital for the correct functioning of the immune system; we cannot expect to be healthy if the immune system is weak. It is also vital for increasing neuromuscular function and improving mood, protecting the brain against toxic chemicals and potentially reducing pain.

The Hormone Conclusion

The key message to take home is that all of these vital agents (hormones) are made from one very important component: cholesterol. Our body has been given this life-giving substance to enable the body to perform its life-giving functions, in other words, to keep us alive and healthy. Where is the logic in blocking or inhibiting this precious substance with a CLD, with all of its side effects, deleterious or otherwise?

9. A NEW, SAFE AND EFFECTIVE WAY TO TREAT HYPERCHOLESTEROLEMIA: THE HORMONODEFICIT HYPOTHESIS

A New Hypothesis to Normalize Cholesterol Levels

We have mentioned normalized cholesterol levels a few times throughout this book. Now it's time to explain the core concept of this statement and how Dr Dzugan's unique hypothesis to normalize cholesterol levels works.

It is important to understand that the aim of this hypothesis is to normalize cholesterol levels rather than to lower them – normalization is the key word! Dr Dzugan prefers to avoid the term 'lowering of cholesterol levels' since low cholesterol, as a static variable, is not something he wants to achieve.

The term used for Dr Dzugan's hypothesis of hypercholesterolemia and its treatment is 'hormonodeficit hypothesis' because the majority of hypercholesterolemia occurs due to an age-related decline in steroid-hormone production or steroidopenia (literally, the deficiency of steroid hormones).

The core concept of hypercholesterolemia is quite simple: cholesterol levels increase when hormone levels decrease – this is a 'cause-and-effect' setup. The cause is the decline in hormones levels and the effect (overall outcome) is an increase in cholesterol levels.

Cholesterol is the precursor to all steroid hormones and is a very significant marker or a 'teller of truths' to what is going on in the body. We know that for every natural hormone there are enzymes (remember, enzymes are special chemicals that speed up the body's processes); hormones cannot be manufactured without the help of these specific enzymes. As the body ages, enzyme reactions become slower and begin to malfunction, therefore the amount of hormones cannot be produced in the same quantities as they were. In short, the malfunctioning enzymes create a decline in hormone production.

As a compensatory mechanism or reaction, the body increases the amount of cholesterol to try and increase hormone production. Unfortunately, this is not the way out – the problem is not the amount of cholesterol but the vast chain of further interconversions. When one link in the chain is broken, we get a breakdown. The body is attempting to fix a broken supply line (but can't do so, as the crucial enzymes are malfunctioning) by increasing the major product (cholesterol). Try as it might, it is unable to do so because the machinery is out of order – it is missing those very important enzymes for the conversion of those very important hormones. In short, hypercholesterolemia is a reactive consequence of an enzyme-dependent down regulation of the creation of steroid hormones and their interconversions.

Although this new hypothesis is actually biologically extremely complex, it is very easy to grasp and makes total sense when it is written down in plain English: steroid-hormone levels fall > cholesterol production increases > steroid hormones are restored (with the use of bioidentical hormones) > cholesterol levels normalize (as they won't have any reason to stay elevated). When cholesterol levels are normalized, the body then functions at its best – optimal. This is what this new hypothesis is all about. Normalization of cholesterol levels!

Practical Application

Following Dr Dzugan's method, normal cholesterol levels are achieved when steroid hormones and cholesterol levels are in the same range as they were during the age interval of twenty to thirty years old. As we mentioned previously, this is the time in life when the production of steroid hormones is at its peak (average age: twenty-five) in a healthy adult and cholesterol production is at its most stable, which would be due to the fact that steroid hormones are at peak production – it is a continual feedback mechanism.

The normalization of cholesterol levels is not a 'one-size-fits-all' approach; it is part of a multimodal and intricate program that targets each person as an individual, not as a unit broken down into variables and statistics. The cholesterol levels of one person are not going to be identical to those of another. Approaching both individuals with the same treatment is not what this hypothesis is about. The 'factory-line' approach is not an optimal solution. 'Normalized', in Dr Dzugan's books (and, of course, in mine as well), stands for the cholesterol levels each individual human being needs to achieve for the body to run and function at optimum – normalized to the levels they had in their healthiest prime, which equals optimal health. To obtain an ideal or normalized cholesterol level, we have to look at each individual and understand where their levels are coming from. We have to look at their physiology. We take an in-depth look at intricate and specific blood tests of steroid-hormone levels, together with a clinical history questionnaire.

Optimizing Hormones, Normalizing Cholesterol

To repeat ourselves, we need to understand that we are all unique and that there is not one person who will have the same cholesterol levels as another even if, let's say, they are given the exact same dosage of bioidentical hormones (which very rarely happens because everyone requires a different dosage of various bioidentical hormones, as determined by blood tests). This is because everyone has his or her unique and individualized physiology. We are all special; we are not a statistic!

Let's take a look at an example: a sixty-three-year-old man joined the program (we will explain more about the program later) with a total cholesterol-level value of 349 mg/dL; at the follow-up blood test, his value was 128 mg/dL. Another lady, aged thirty-nine, came in at 202 mg/dL; at the follow-up blood test, her value was 164 mg/dL. Other values range from 232 mg/dL to 198 mg/dL for a fifty-three-year-old female, and 221 mg/dL to 190 mg/dL for an eighty-two-year-old male. These results do not mean that one outcome was more successful than another, but what it is showing us is that each individual has his or her own unique or individualized physiology. We are all special, not a statistic or variable that's been hung out to dry!

Here we feel we need to make a distinction between low and normalized cholesterol levels as you may have found the discussion related to the sixty-three-year-old man somewhat confusing. His levels normalized at 128 mg/dL from 349 mg/dL, which can be considered quite a big drop. We have said time and time again that a low level of cholesterol is not good because of increased mortality and all the health issues that go with it. Low levels of cholesterol by default are bad because they are a marker for low steroid-hormone production.

But here comes the distinction. We are not talking about a level that has been achieved by way of a cholesterol-lowering drug but by restoring hormone levels to optimal with the safe use of bioidentical hormones. This is a totally different concept. When you block the cholesterol-making pathway, at the same time you interfere with the pathway that makes hormones, hormones that are already low due to the aging process and the malfunction of crucial enzymes. CLDs lower hormone production even further, exacerbating the situation. On the other hand, when we restore and optimize low hormone levels, the root issue and warning signs and/or malaise associated with low cholesterol levels is rectified because these health issues are, in fact, the outcome (effect) of low steroid hormones. As such, this new low level (or, rather, normalized level) of cholesterol is associated with healthy and optimal steroid-hormone production, as reflected in the values we had in our 'prime time' during the twenty to thirty age bracket. This is the normalized level for that specific person, not an actual lowered level. This is in direct opposition to the low levels attained by CLDs which lower cholesterol and, at the same time, keep steroid-hormone production low. Not a good idea. We reiterate: we are all different; we are not a statistic!

Let's take this from another angle: if an individual's cholesterol, which we will call 'A', is lowered by 80 mg/dL, and another individual's cholesterol, which we will call 'B', is lowered by 30 mg/dL, it by no way means that 'A' got a more satisfactory result than 'B'. They both got the desired result, i.e. they both achieved normalized cholesterol levels for that individual's physiology. And, in fact, on observing lab data (hormone status), individual 'B' may well have a better hormone profile than 'A'. In no way, manner or form can cholesterol have a static association with hormone production. As we mentioned previously, each body works differently; we all regulate, metabolize and use hormones differently – this, of course, will have a feedback effect on cholesterol synthesis. It will determine how much cholesterol is needed at a specific time and for that individual. It is the hormonal production that dictates the amount of cholesterol we need. And it is how we regulate, metabolize and use these hormones that dictates our physiology.

Another reason why we prefer to use 'normalization' rather than 'lowering' of cholesterol is because not all cholesterol levels need to be lowered. To explain: the hypothesis of hypercholesterolemia can be turned around into hypocholesterolemia. In the latter, low cholesterol levels are the cause of low steroid production (there is not enough cholesterol to go around). Of course, in this case we certainly wouldn't want to lower cholesterol levels. However, here's the good part – we can't! In both cases (hyper- and hypocholesterolemia) we are restoring hormone levels to optimal levels (the range we had at twenty to thirty years old). In other words, restoring steroid-hormone levels in the case of hypercholesterolemia lowers the levels of cholesterol because there is no need for extra cholesterol production. In the case of hypocholesterolemia we are restoring the hormone levels which are low and are the underlying issue at hand. To use an analogy, cholesterol is, in both cases, a thermostat. This approach works to fix the temperature but not break the thermostat – by correcting the temperature at both levels, the desired effect is achieved.

A Look at Steroid Hormones and Their Effect on Cholesterol

The effects of estrogens and androgens were first looked at in the early 1900s. Estrogens were synthetically created in the 1920s largely to help alleviate menopausal symptoms and, at that time, even to reduce ischemic cardiovascular disease. Androgens have been studied and written about since 1936 and were found to relieve vasomotor (the widening and narrowing of blood vessels) symptoms in menopausal women. Recently performed studies show that a combination of androgen and estrogen therapy reduced levels of total cholesterol, LDL, HDL and triglycerides. DHEA as a single supplement, which was bioidentical to the human hormone, was also seen to reduce total cholesterol and LDL. However, various other studies failed to confirm these observations.

Apart from Dr Dzugan's many published articles, up until the last decade there was no medical literature that presented a connection between the restoration of youthful levels of steroid hormones and the normalization of cholesterol. Over the last twenty years, Dr Dzugan has published twenty-five articles on this topic alone.

The Controversy: Steroid Hormones and the Correction of Lipid Disorders

There has been a lot of controversy in the media about steroid hormones and the correction of lipid disorders, which is largely due to studies done using DHEA and androgens, as well as estrogens and progesterone (considered hormone replacement therapy (HRT), not hormone restorative therapy). HRT does not in any way begin to balance or restore hormones. And it certainly does not offer sufficient or adequate levels of hormones, nor are the hormones used bioidentical or given in the correct physiological dosage. In most cases hormone use in hormone replacement therapy follows a 'one-size-fits-all' regime with the use of one or two standardized hormones. The very significant and important difference in absorption rate, metabolism and preexisting hormone levels in each individual body is totally missed and not even considered! And, in fact, this is exactly where the failure rate for hypercholesterolemia and steroid hormones comes in, in connection with HRT.

Dr Dzugan believes that the majority of treatments have failed because only one or two hormones were utilized when, in fact, what was needed was multiple bioidentical-hormone administration to correct and normalize cholesterol levels. When the 'human network of health' is restored to youthful hormone levels, and therefore optimized, cholesterol will also be normalized. To achieve normalized cholesterol levels, **all** hormones must be adequately restored and precisely balanced within their respective ratios to get the desired results. In other words, the safe and efficient correction of hypercholesterolemia is achievable only when all hormones are restored to youthful levels. This, of course, is not something that Dr Dzugan has just pulled out of thin air but from a myriad of clinical evidence that supports his hypothesis. He has his own scientific data to reinforce his hypothesis; he has everything that is needed to support his claims – scientific data!

The primary difference between hormone restorative therapy and conventional treatments (CLDs), which deliberately and directly decrease cholesterol levels by interfering with a bodily mechanism, is that hormone restorative medicine does not go all out to lower cholesterol levels but achieves normalized levels (which is actually a lowered, but to healthy and safe, level for that person) through a multitude of natural feedback mechanisms related to youthful hormone levels, in an indirect fashion (steroid hormones are increased while cholesterol is decreased).

To explain further: low hormone production affects the compensatory mechanism to increase the production of cholesterol through multiple feedback actions which try, through a combined effort, to restore homeostasis by increasing production of the precursor (cholesterol). Statins inhibit the natural production of cholesterol and, therefore, cause a further decrease in steroid-hormone production, which can cause multiple unwanted health consequences. The inhibition of extra cholesterol synthesis, which naturally occurs to offset declining steroid-hormone production during aging, leads to somatic, psychological and immune impairment. This includes decreased defense against cancer and infections, as well as the speeding up of the aging process with various noncardiovascular disorders and a loss of quality of life!

Hormone restorative therapy, on the other hand, normalizes cholesterol levels in a safe, efficient and natural way, without decreasing hormone production. Hormonorestorative therapy offers us all-over quality of life, protects against disease and illnesses, and slows the aging process.

Relative Hypercholesterolemia and Familial Hypercholesterolemia
Included in Dr Dzugan's hypothesis are the 'relative' and 'familial' types of hypercholesterolemia. These are two very important ideas that were formed in the process of observing the results of patients on the program.

Relative Hypercholesterolemia

To explain: let's look at a fifty-four-year-old woman with initial total cholesterol levels of 170 mg/dL; at her follow-up blood test this value dropped to 140 mg/dL. This initial value, of course, cannot be considered hypercholesterolemia and, in fact, is quite a long stretch away from the lowest range to enable it to be labeled as such. It is interesting to note that this particular woman did not join the program with the intent of lowering her cholesterol levels but, rather, to optimize her health status. The lowering of her cholesterol level was a consequence of hormone optimization. It was only after hormone levels had been optimized that this new level of cholesterol was achieved.

In short, even though the initial level of cholesterol was normal, it was 'high' in relation to the level of cholesterol that would have been present at a youthful or peak age of optimal (for her) steroid-hormone production. The 'relative' part of this hypothesis is key since it is relative to the original number (170 mg/dL), which definitely cannot be considered hypercholesterolemia. In other words, it is relative to that individual person, not to some scientific vote that boosts sales for the pharmaceutical industry. It is important to understand that life-cycle elevation of total cholesterol is a vital component to understanding what is going on with cholesterol and steroid-hormone metabolism.

In fact, Dr Dzugan firmly believes that, because steroid hormones decline with age and cholesterol levels then rise, it is much more important to look at cholesterol elevation over an individual's lifetime rather than see an isolated level with little context. Observing how steroid-hormone levels decline over time can show the risk for disease in a far better manner than one or two inefficient tests for a cholesterol value in the short term. The table below shows a perfect example of the difference between relative hypercholesterolemia and regular hypercholesterolemia:

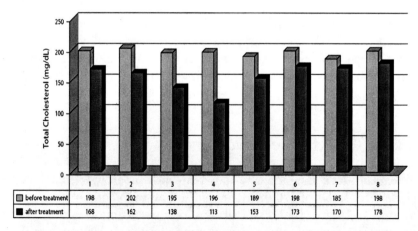

	1	2	3	4	5	6	7	8
before treatment	198	202	195	196	189	198	185	198
after treatment	168	162	138	113	153	173	170	178

Relative Hypercholsterolemia
Total Cholesterol Before and After Hormonorestorative Therapy

Age	25	40
Patient 1 Total cholesterol (nl – 200 mg/dL)	130	190
Patient 2 Total cholesterol (nl – 200 mg/dL)	180	240

The first patient is relative hypercholesterolemia, while the second is regular hypercholesterolemia.

Familial Hypercholesterolemia

Familial hypercholesterolemia (FHC) is a frequently inherited disorder which is characterized by elevated levels of total cholesterol and LDL and affects one in every 500 people. The general accepted explanation for FHC is that there is a mutation in gene coding for the LDL receptor protein; in other words, these people lack the receptor that identifies LDL. In short, this means that LDL is unable to lock onto their receptors. Therefore, LDL, together with cholesterol, is left 'floating' in the blood and so the amount accumulates to levels higher than they should be. However, based on Dr Dzugan's experience and observations, he has a more detailed explanation for the occurrence of FHC to be explained later!

FHC occurs much more frequently in certain groups of people such as Afrikaners, Christian Lebanese, French Canadians and Ashkenazi Jews. One explanation could be that people from these groups tended to migrate and found new colonies. In other words, certain groups tend to marry and reproduce within the same groups, therefore they will have children who are more likely to carry gene mutations. However, FHC has a strong association with environmental factors as well, not just genetics.

There is no doubt that FHC has health risks attached to it as it has been associated with an increased frequency of coronary heart disease, with the worst outcome being heart attack at an early age and premature death. Life expectancy in people with this mutant gene is reduced by fifteen to thirty years unless they are treated with therapy to lower lipid levels. It is, therefore, advisable for individuals with a family history of FHC, or significantly elevated cholesterol or heart disease, to be tested to see if FHC is present.

A standard physical examination can reveal and identify these details: Xanthomas, which are yellowish firm nodules in the skin lesions caused by cholesterol-rich lipoprotein deposits.

Xanthelasmas, which are very small (1 mm-2 mm) yellowish plaques that are slightly raised on the skin surface of the upper or lower eyelid. Arcus senilis cornea, which is a whitish discoloration of the iris.

Meanwhile, laboratory testing may show these details:

- Total plasma cholesterol that is greater than 300 mg/dL in adults.
- Total plasma cholesterol that is greater than 250 mg/dL in children.
- An LDL level that is higher than 200 mg/dL, as well as elevated triglycerides.
- Protein electrophoresis (a process to determine protein amounts) may show abnormal results.

An LDL receptor gene defect can be identified with genetic testing.

Even though billions of dollars are being invested in the research and development of many cholesterol-lowering drugs, coronary heart disease is still the leading 'killer' in developed countries and FHC is a major contributing factor to this deadly killer.

There are various options that may help with the management of FHC: a diet low in saturated fats, cholesterol-lowering medication, daily exercise, weight control, and cessation of smoking. These options may help prevent deposits in the skin, thickening of the Achilles tendon, atherosclerosis and premature death. Of course, other options include the statin drug; since its introduction in 1986, the treatment of FHC has improved but, more often than not, statin drugs alone are not enough and additional treatments such as the recently invented (July 2015) PCSK9 inhibitors (of which we spoke in chapter 4) are offered. Remember that the outcome on cardiovascular mortality and morbidity has not yet been established for these drugs and that larger and long-term studies are needed to determine their safety and efficiency. Other treatments consist of Vytorin which was approved by the FDA in 2004. This drug is a compound formula, specifically targeting FHC. Vytorin is a combination of ezetimibe (which inhibits cholesterol absorption in the intestinal tract) and simvastatin (which inhibits the creation of cholesterol) – a 'two-way' attack method. The long-term effect of ezetimibe is still unknown with regards to FHC, cardiovascular morbidity and mortality. And, of course, there is still the discussion about the many serious side effects associated with the statin drug: poor quality of life, severe rhabdomyolysis, renal failure, death, and many more issues.

We already know that statins present many, many health issues but what is even more concerning is the long-term use in our precious children that has not yet been established. Long-term exposure to these drugs may affect growth and sexual development – knowing what we know and the mechanisms of cholesterol, this seems more than obvious. Remember, statins decrease cholesterol biosynthesis and, therefore, the production of hormones which are so vital to both mental and physical growth and repair.

Recall our discussion of the significant increase in cholesterol levels in pregnant women, which would be due to an increased need of hormones for both baby and mother. This reflects how sensitive the body is to its requirements. The body is so efficient that it reacts immediately by increasing the production of cholesterol when there is an increased demand for hormones.

One study showed that DHEA-S levels were reduced in both girls and boys who took a statin drug as opposed to those treated with a placebo. Even a small change in hormonal production at a young age can lead to major problems in adult life. Think about this one, please!

Is Familial Hypercholesterolemia a Resolvable Issue?

Yes! From Dr Dzugan's experience, he believes it is. From his observations of individuals suffering from FHC and high cholesterol, he found that, when their hormone levels were balanced and optimized, their cholesterol levels normalized. The results were extremely encouraging, to say the least, and, importantly, came without any of the side effects (dangerous or otherwise) that are so prevalent with cholesterol-lowering drugs.

Dr Dzugan believes that FHC works with the same mechanism as age-related cholesterol elevation does – the 'malfunctioning-enzyme' phenomena. It is a compensatory reaction of low steroid-hormone production due to a congenital defect of the enzyme system that is responsible for the regulation of the biosynthesis of steroid hormones and their interconversions. In other words, individuals with FHC have the same defects in the enzymatic system that controls cholesterol metabolism, starting from birth, as those seen in the body as it ages.

Again, this malfunction of the enzyme systems leads to a diminished ability to produce basic steroid hormones, regardless of the overproduction of cholesterol. This situation naturally leads to hypercholesterolemia – it is a normal feedback mechanism where hormone deficiency serves as the 'starting point' for the overproduction of cholesterol. When there is low steroid-hormone production, there will be an increase in cholesterol production – this is something that goes without saying. The body is trying to maintain homeostasis.

When there is a high synthesis of cholesterol, there will be an excess of LDL in the blood (remember, LDL is the primary plasma carrier and delivery service of cholesterol from the liver to the tissues, or parts of the body, where it is then absorbed by the cells of the body and used as needed). It is an automatic feedback mechanism – the body needs to do its job correctly and deliver the agent to the appropriate tissues/ organs throughout the body and to keep the infrastructure up and running correctly. However, the body will not increase the number of LDL receptors on the cell surface as there is no need because hormone production is low (because of enzyme malfunction). Under normal circumstances, in a healthy functioning body the LDL would attach itself to the LDL receptor, which then releases cholesterol into the cells to be converted into pregnenolone and a cascade of other steroid hormones to be used appropriately. When there are not enough receptor sites to manage, disperse or cope with the influx of cholesterol, this will obviously lead to an excess flow of LDL in the blood.

It seems, however, and not so remarkably (remember, the body is very logical and very, very clever), that the body purposely produces less LDL receptors as a defense mechanism against high cholesterol. If this process were not to happen, rather large amounts of cholesterol would be deposited into the cells without the ability to use them for hormone production (as they could not be converted into pregnenolone, and the following cascade, due to the malfunction of enzymes). The cells would then become overloaded with cholesterol which in turn may block, and would certainly disturb, normal cell function. This overload of cholesterol in the cells is exactly what we are seeing with the 'revolutionary' (a touch of sarcasm here) PCSK9 inhibitors.

If you recall, PCSK9 inhibitors work by blocking the PCSK enzyme, which allows more LDL receptors on the cell surface to be produced, which in turn allows for more LDL cholesterol to be absorbed into the cells. The outcome is that the cells will be totally overloaded with cholesterol, which is not a natural event. The body does not have the correct infrastructure to deal with such a setup. Our cells do not know what to do with this large amount of cholesterol which cannot be converted into hormones. This drug messes with cell function and more than likely will cause all types of dysfunction in the body. Not good!

So What Is FHC?

Dr Dzugan believes that FHC should not be viewed as the primary disease (in that the main theme is the increased production of cholesterol), rather, as a secondary disorder connected to a problem with the biosynthesis of steroid hormones. Therefore, familial hypercholesterolemia would become familial low steroidal hormone production. Patients who followed the hormonorestorative therapy (HT) program stood true to Dr Dzugan's hypothesis: when hormones were restored to youthful and healthy levels, their total cholesterol and LDL levels normalized.

The Last Remark on Hypercholesterolemia

And here we have arrived at the last remark on hypercholesterolemia. At this point we would like to share with you another very important and interesting piece of information: Dr Dzugan believes that there is yet another way to normalize cholesterol-level physiology without the use of CLD – 'enzymes' is the key word here. Enzymes, as we already know, control the down regulation of steroid biosynthesis and, with age or because of a genetic error, can become damaged and/or dysfunction. However, these damaged or malfunctioning enzymes can be replaced fairly easily. The P450scc (cholesterol desmolase) enzyme, for example, can be used for catalyzing (a chemical reaction that sets in motion) the conversion of cholesterol to pregnenolone. Also, the combination of other enzymes (such as P450c17 (17 alpha-hydroxylase/17,20-lyase) and P450c21 (21-hydroxylase), 11beta- and 18-hydroxylase, etc.) can normalize the process of steroidogenesis (production of steroids) and further levels of steroid biosynthesis. There is no doubt that this approach is extremely promising. For more than twenty years Dr Dzugan has strived to make this possible but, unfortunately, supplement companies don't have any interest in producing these enzymes because there is no money to be made; enzymes are very cheap to produce but the process for FDA approval is very, very expensive. No big-profit margins in this direction. Such a simple and logical solution, yet seeming so unreachable. Very sad.

Optimized Physiology: How We Get There

We have spoken many times throughout this book about optimal health. It is now time to discuss exactly what the program consists of and, through this, how an optimal health status is achieved for each individual. The program begins with two fundamental cores: a client health history and initial blood tests. The client health history is laid out in a way as to obtain as much information about the health of the client (both past and present) with, of course, different areas for both men and women. The questions asked allow Dr Dzugan to gauge the health status of the individual and give him a clear guide as to what is, or has been, going on in the client's body.

A client health history allows the client to relay any major or minor health issues they may have: starting from less life-destroying symptoms such as hot flashes in both men and women (yes, men have them too), brittle nails and hair, hair loss, weight gain, acne, low stress resilience, depression, mood swings, fatigue, low libido, poor digestion; to the more soul-destroying issues (which would be classed as a chronic disease state) such as heart disease, cancer, diabetes, eye diseases (macular degeneration and cataracts), and many more. Symptoms speak volumes. The less life-destroying symptoms are telling you what's to come; it is your body talking, telling you that, if you don't correct these initial niggling symptoms, the worst is yet to come, i.e. chronic disease!

This, together with specific blood tests, gives Dr Dzugan a complete understanding of the client's health to date. As an example, the initial case history of a woman who is suffering hot flashes may seem to suggest that progesterone supplementation is advisable but, until the precise progesterone value has been observed against estrogen(s) values (recall our discussion on estrogen or progesterone dominance, as the case may be), the exact dosage of progesterone cannot be recommended. As an example, it could be that levels of estrogen are relatively high (compared to progesterone) or relatively low (but progesterone is lower still), so both would be classed as estrogen dominance. It is the blood tests that give him the precise missing piece of the puzzle for dosage recommendation. Restorative medicine is an art, a very precise medicine that has the accuracy and ability to take us to the realms of optimal health.

Blood Tests

For the creation of an individualized program, the blood tests Dr Dzugan asks for are listed below, with follow-up blood tests at three months, six months and one year, or more frequently if necessary. Thereafter, blood tests can be done at yearly intervals once optimization of physiology is achieved.

Complete Blood Count (CBC)

This test offers important information about the types and numbers of cells in the blood. A CBC assists Dr Dzugan in diagnosing different conditions and issues, allowing us to see if there is a dysfunction of the immune system and other factors such as coagulation. This test covers issues such as erythrocytes (red blood cells, which are the most common type of blood cells and are responsible for the delivery of oxygen to the body tissue), lymphocytes (a type of white blood cell that increases in number in response to viral infections), platelets (cell fragments which are responsible for clotting action), hemoglobin (iron-carrying proteins), etc.

Comprehensive Metabolic Panel (CMP)

A range of tests which assist in understanding an individual's physiology. They include general tests such as glucose and calcium, as well as tests for electrolytes such as sodium and potassium. A larger part of this test has signifiers for kidney and liver function; examples of these are creatinine (a breakdown product in muscle which is filtered through the kidneys) and ALT (an enzyme which is found in the highest amounts in the liver and is released into the blood when damage to the liver occurs).

Lipid Profile

This test includes the overall cholesterol value, LDL, HDL, triglycerides and VLDL.

Pregnenolone

As pregnenolone is the precursor to other steroid hormones and is essential to creating an individualized program.

DHEA-Sulphate

DHEA-S provides a much more precise value than DHEA for the overall body (for reasons discussed in chapter 8 under 'DHEA').

Total Testosterone

Dr Dzugan prefers to look at total testosterone as opposed to free testosterone. This is because free testosterone may not give the correct values of actual testosterone production. Free testosterone means it is available and unbound, it is floating about; this test does not take into account the testosterone that is chemically bound, therefore numbers may not be accurate. Total testosterone, on the other hand, takes all these factors into account, giving Dr Dzugan a much better overall and accurate account of testosterone levels. Free testosterone numbers may be normal or high when total testosterone levels are actually low.

PSA

This is a prostate-specific antigen, an important protein produced within the prostate that is necessary for optimal function. When there are elevated levels of this protein, this can signify prostate malfunction or cancer.

Total Estrogens

A test for estrogens usually incorporates the three major estrogens: estriol, estradiol and estrone. However, to get an accurate gauge, it is far better to look at all estrogens. If only the major three are focused on, it wouldn't be an efficient method of gauging estrogen production. For women who are still menstruating, the ideal time to take this test is three to seven days prior to the beginning of menses – the fluctuating nature of this level is always considered.

Progesterone

This is a simple test; there are no total or free measurements floating around. Again, the time in the menstruating cycle (if applicable) is also considered.

Cortisol

This stress hormone is an important value to know. Knowing if levels are too high or too low is vital to creating an individualized program.

Aldosterone

This hormone assists the body in regulating blood pressure and has been seen to help with issues such as dizziness, headaches, hearing loss and tinnitus.

Vitamin D3

Vitamin D3 has a significant impact on cholesterol production and, thus, on cholesterol values. Recall our discussion about the creation of vitamin D3 from cholesterol through the action of sunlight (ultraviolet radiation)?

The tests for serotonin, homocysteine, prolactin and C-reactive protein do not have a direct association with the normalization of cholesterol but are part of the individualized program and are essential for the optimization of physiology, which translates into optimal health.

Serotonin

Serotonin, along with norepinephrine, is a major neurotransmitter that controls mood in the brain. When levels of serotonin are low, this may cause depression (remember, we discussed this in chapter 8 under 'Estrogens'). There are numerous drugs on the marketplace to treat depression but, unfortunately, they manipulate this neurotransmitter and can lead to extremely low levels as they become depleted.

Homocysteine

Homocysteine is an amino acid that serves as a marker for cardiovascular disease when levels are high. However, low levels are not optimal either – balance is required for optimal health.

Prolactin

Prolactin has a strong relationship with serotonin, dopamine, thyroid hormone, estrogens, progesterone and testosterone, and it has various functions such as lactation, but is equally important in both men and women. It is not only synthesized in the pituitary gland, as once thought, but also within the central nervous system (CNS), immune system, the uterus and its associated tissues of conception, and even in the mammary gland itself. Its biological actions are not solely concentrated on reproduction as it controls a variety of behaviors and has even been seen to play a role in homeostasis.

C-reactive Protein

When levels of this protein are elevated, they show that inflammation is present in the body.

Once an individual has initiated the program, apart from the follow-up blood tests, Dr Dzugan and his team also monitor the entire process in the form of updates; the more updates, the better – weekly is good. Updates give them that extra information needed to understand the changes that are occurring within the body and to achieve optimal health. Working with and listening to the client is a vital part of achieving the highest results.

Hormonorestorative Therapy Explained

Hormonorestorative therapy is a term Dr Dzugan has used since 1996. It is defined as a multi-hormonal therapy that uses a formula chemically identical to human (bioidentical) hormones and is administered in physiological ratios and dosages that simulate the natural human production cycle, thus allowing hormones to be restored to optimal levels. The recommended doses are determined by clinical data, serum-hormone levels and the so-called 'optimal range' – the latter is defined as a level of hormones in one-third of the highest normal range for all steroid hormones of healthy individuals aged between twenty and thirty. This precise and cutting-edge therapy enables Dr Dzugan to restore hormone levels to optimum. It is the 'golden key' to the program. However, the program is not solely based on hormones as there are various supplements and agents that interact with hormones and assist hormone activity.

As an example, zinc has been seen to play an important role in modulating and increasing serum testosterone in normal men. Another would be saw palmetto that prevents the conversion of testosterone into dihydrotestosterone (DHT); DHT is a much more powerful form of testosterone but offers side effects such as hair loss, prostate enlargement and acne. As men age, levels of testosterone decrease and the body can then go into panic mode by attempting to correct this deficiency by converting a weaker testosterone into a stronger one (DHT). However, the side effects of too much DHT are less than favorable, one of which includes prostate issues. Another agent would be omega-3 fatty acids, otherwise known as fish oils (although krill oil is preferable as it contains a phospholipid complex that increases absorption), which can assist in lowering triglyceride levels.

Cholesterol as an Optimal Marker for the Aging Process

Dr Dzugan believes that the changing level of cholesterol is the perfect marker of the aging process and a good tool to approximate the best time an individual should initiate hormonorestorative therapy. Again, cholesterol is the 'teller of truths'! Hypercholesterolemia is the evidence that the body is dysfunctioning and homeostasis is bobbing around in rough waters. Dr Dzugan believes that elevated levels of total cholesterol (including relative hypercholesterolemia), and particularly when they are joined with steroidopenia (deficient hormonal levels), are an excellent marker for the restoration of hormonal levels (levels that existed in our youth).

Optimal levels of steroid hormones such as pregnenolone, DHEA, progesterone, estrogens, vitamin D3, cortisol and testosterone in the correct ratios are required to achieve and maintain an optimal health status for both men and women. As you have understood from our discussion on hormones in chapter 8, hormones are responsible for an array of vital physiological functions, and the alteration, decline and/or imbalance of these levels play a key role in how we age – in sickness or in health; how we confront life – with positivity or negativity; who we are – vital, strong and healthy; and how long we live.

Summarizing What Really Causes Atherosclerosis

Based on the information you have just read, we hope you have a much clearer and far better understanding of what cholesterol truly is and what really does cause atherosclerosis. We hope we have clarified that it is not, in fact, cholesterol that is the prime suspect in heart disease. Rather, it is our daily savior, having many all-over functions in the body, one of which is to act as a key component in the repair process.

Cholesterol Is a Key Component of the Repair Process

Cholesterol is not the 'start' of the breakdown process but the 'end' product of degeneration. In other words, cholesterol is part of a healing process (of the initial scratch, microtrauma or wound) that has been caused by something else, such as high blood pressure, excess triglycerides, low blood EPA/DHA (Omega-3s), elevated C-reactive Protein, oxidized LDL particles, high glucose, nitric oxide deficit, low vitamin K, excess insulin, excess fibrinogen (clot-promoting substance), excess homocysteine, low testosterone and excessively high cholesterol levels. It is the actual initial damage or injury to the endothelium that instigates the healing process, provoking an accumulation of various powerful healing materials such as cholesterol and, as a scar-like tissue forms, a high content of cholesterol appears. Cholesterol is vital to the normal process of tissue repair; every cell membrane and organelle within the cells is rich in cholesterol.

Atherosclerosis is a consequence of an age-related shift from anabolic (build-up) to catabolic (breakdown) process which slowly leads to tissue degeneration. Age provokes a 'body-breakdown' situation. When the body breaks down, there is a loss of regenerative capacity which brings with it an accumulation of cellular damage. The aging process creates a 'seesaw' setup between damage and repair; this can be seen at every level, from the DNA to the cells, organs and the entire body. The speed at which we age depends on the ratio between damage and repair. Repair, rebuild and regenerate are generally described as anabolic. Instead, the damage we experience and accumulate over time is termed catabolic. Hormonal loss, environmental pollution, highly processed foods, ultraviolet radiation, dehydration, stress, obesity and a sedentary lifestyle are all catabolic accelerators.

When catabolic influences overpower anabolic influences within the human metabolism, our hearts are left less protected. The breakdown and build-up process becomes imbalanced, in other words, the heart is not capable of repairing itself fast enough or adequately enough, which in turn will lead to an incomplete healing process. The overall interpretation of this is that atherosclerosis is a physical adaptation to vascular injury (that was initiated by a microtrauma or scratch) and is part of a failed healing process due to body breakdown without enough repair.

Dr Dzugan believes that the main reason for atherosclerosis is a dominance of catabolic processes which start after the age of thirty and slowly increase. The race is now on. The question is – who will run the fastest for the longest: anabolic or catabolic metabolism? Which one will maintain a greater hold on the aging process? If we don't at least try to control it, the catabolic process will always win.

The building-up (anabolic) and tearing-down (catabolic) effects are both essential for a healthy body; however, both have to be correctly balanced. Hormones play a critical role between damage and repair because they are the most comprehensive messaging machine in the human body. When hormones are restored, they will balance the damaging process and the race of life will be easier. The 'seesaw' will be tipped in your favor, helping to support the repair function throughout the body, the heart and the brain. It is all to do with the physiology of the human body. Regenerating our capacity for repair and reducing cellular damage is key to a long and healthy life. Age is a vicious cycle: the older we get, the faster we age because there is more damage and less repair. Damage with little repair. When you restore your body, you protect yourself and your heart! No more cholesterol-lowering drugs needed.

CONCLUSION

So you got to your final destination and, of course, you are happy, right? You now have the solution to preventing and treating heart disease and, at the same time, you have a safe and efficient way to obtain positive longevity. You have learnt about cholesterol and its connection to hormone production, as well as the impact each hormone has on your body. You have learnt that hormones decline with age and that they are powerful molecules that keep the immune system strong, keep us safe, health, vibrant, positive, sexy, sensual and energetic.

You have now understood what cholesterol truly is: not the 'causer' of heart disease you were led to believe it was! You now no longer feel you 'have to' take those devastating statin drugs to protect you from heart disease or a heart attack. You now know that there is a natural, healthy, safe and efficient alternative out there for resolving hypercholesterolemia and protecting your heart and general health. You now understand what normalized cholesterol levels are and how important they are to overall health. You now have the information needed to take control of your own life. You are happy. We can see you smiling. We are happy too!

You have now understood that cholesterol is a vitally important component of the body and, without it, the body would be unable to function correctly. We are happy because you are happy. You have now understood that cholesterol does not start the actual process of atherosclerosis, rather, it is the end product of degeneration – it is a repair molecule. You are no longer afraid of the word 'cholesterol'. You have understood what it means: a molecule of abundant health, repair and regeneration.

You have learnt that steroidopenia (a deficiency of steroid hormones) is central to the mechanism of hypercholesterolemia; when hormones decline, cholesterol levels rise.

You have learnt that cholesterol can be used as a marker of physiological function or dysfunction, that it is a perfect marker of your health, an indicator that the body is either functioning correctly or incorrectly. Cholesterol is the 'teller of truths'. You have learnt that hypercholesterolemia not only reflects a serious problem with steroidal hormone production but serves as an excellent marker which can be used to define the time when a patient should begin hormonorestorative therapy.

You have learnt that the purpose of cholesterol elevation is to increase production of steroid hormones and vitamin D3; to repair damaged cell structure (membrane); to heal a damaged endothelium by the 'plaquing' of tears and holes; and to provide a normal response to physiologic demand (growth, pregnancy, stress, starvation, etc.).

You have learnt, however, that an extremely high level of cholesterol can lead to vascular damage with stenosis or occlusion of arteries, if the reason or 'the why' for cholesterol elevation is not corrected in time. You have learnt that CLDs are not the correct way to go about correcting cholesterol levels; CLDs do not correct 'the why' cholesterol levels rise ('the why' being steroidal hormone decline), instead, they fight the consequence or outcome (i.e. high cholesterol) and not the real cause of hypercholesterolemia. CLDs do not resolve anything, they make the situation worse; they cannot resolve as they miss the point of origin ('the why') and have no physiological foundation to enable them to offer a solution to hypercholesterolemia.

Importantly, you have learnt about the new hypothesis of hypercholesterolemia which implies that the elevation of cholesterol is the compensatory mechanism in the decline of steroidal hormone production.

You have learnt about hormonorestorative therapy and it being an effective strategy for maintaining cholesterol homeostasis in patients who have hypercholesterolemia and sub-youthful serum steroidal hormones. You have learnt so much. You have learnt that hormonorestoration is typically associated with a substantial drop in serum TC (total cholesterol) and is, without doubt, a physiologic and inexpensive resource for the healthcare system.

REFERENCES

Chapter 1

Miedema MD, Lopez FL, Blaha MJ, Virani SS, Coresh J, et al. Eligibility for Statin Therapy According to New Cholesterol Guidelines and Prevalent Use of Medication to Lower Lipid Levels in an Older US Cohort. The Atherosclerosis Risk in Communities Study Cohort. JAMA Intern Med. 2015; 175(1):138-140.

Starfield B. Is US health really the best in the world? JAMA. 2000; 284(4):483-5.

Smith D. Cardiovascular disease: a history perspective. Jpn J Vet Res. 2000; 48(2-3):147-66.

Jacobson TA. Clincial context: current concepts of coronary heart disease management. Am J Med. 2001; 110 Suppl 6A:3S-11S.

Bolland MJ, Grey A, Avenell A, Gamble GD, Reid IR. Calcium supplements with or without vitamin D and risk of cardiovascular events: reanalysis of the Women's Health Initiative limited access dataset and meta-analysis. BMJ. 2011 Apr 19; 342:d2040. doi: 10.1136/bmj.d2040.

Widman L, Wester PO, Stegmayr BK, Wirell M. The dose-dependent reduction in blood pressure through administration of magnesium. A double blind placebo controlled cross-over study. Am J Hypertens. 1993 Jan; 6(1):41-5.

Virchow, R (1856). Phlogose und Thrombose im Gefassystem. In: Gesammelte Abhandlungen zurwissenschaftlichen Medizin. Germany: Staatsdruckerei Frankfurt.

Tshudi MR, Noll G, Lusher TP. Pharmacotherapy of arteriosclerosis and its complications. Efffects of ACE inhibitors and HMG-CoA-reductase inhibitors. Schweiz Med Wochenschr. 1997 Apr 12; 127(15):636-49.

Kaunitz H. The significance of dietary fat in arteriosclerosis. An outmoded theory? MMW Munch Wochenschr. 1997 Apr 12; 119(16):539-42.

Chapter 2

Bjorkhem I, Meaney S. Brain cholesterol: long secret life behind a barrier. Arterioscler Thromb Vasc Biol. 2004 May; 24(5):806-15.

Vance JE, Hayashi H, Karten B. Cholesterol homeostasis in neurons and glial cells. Semin Cell Dev Biol. 2005 Apr; 16(2):193-212.

Lythgoe C, Perkes A, Peterson M, Schmutz C, Leary M, Ebbert MT, et al. Population-based analysis of cholesteryl ester transfer protein identifies association between 1405V and cognitive decline: the Cache County Study. Neurobiol Aging. 2015 Jan; 36(1):547.

Pfrieger F. Brain Researcher Discovers Bright Side of 111-famed Molecule. Science, 9 November, 2001.

Koudinova NV, Berezov TT, Koudinov AR. Cholesterol failure is a unifying cause of neurodegeneration. Neurobiol.Lipids. 2004; 3:7.

Koudinov AR, Koudinova NV. Cholesterol homeostasis failure as a unifying cause of synaptic degeneration. J Neurol Sci. 2005 Mar 15; 229-230,233-40.

Flegel WA, et al. Inhibition of Endotoxin-Induced Activation of Human Monocytes by Human Lipoproteins, Infection and Immunity 57. No. 7 (1989):2237-45.

Flegel WA, et al. Prevention of Endotoxin-Induced Monokine Released by Human Low- and High- Density Lipoproteins and by Apolipoprotein A-1, Infection and Immunity 61. No., 12 (1993):5140-46.

Flegel WA, Wolpl A, Mannel DN, Northoff H. Inhibition of endotoxin-induced activation of human monocytes by human lipoproteins. Infect Immun.1989 Jul; 57(7):2237-45.

Calvo MS, Whiting SJ, Barton CN. Vitamin D intake, A global perspective of current status. J Nutr. 2007; 135:310-17.

Dr Zahid MBBS, DPH, FCPS, Professor. Vitamin D Deficiency – An Ignored Epidemic. Int J Health Sci (Qassim). 2010 Jan; 4(1):V-VI.

Chapter 3

Jacobs DR Jr, Irribarren C. Invited commentary: low cholesterol and nonatherosclerotic disease risk: a persistently perplexing question. Am J Epidemiol. 2000 Apr 15; 151(8):748-51.

Elshourbagy NA, Meyers HV, Abdel-Meguid SS. Cholesterol: the good, the bad, and the ugly – therapeutic targets for the treatment of dyslipidemia. Med Princ Pract. 2014; 23(2):99-11.

Chapter 4

Virchow, R (1856). Phlogose und Thrombose im Gefassystem. In: Gesammelte Abhandlungen zurwissenschaftlichen Medizin. Germany: Staatsdruckerei Frankfurt.

Clarkson S, Newburgh LH. The relation between Atherosclerosis and Ingested cholesterol in the rabbit. J Exp Med. 1926 Apr 30; 43(5):595-612.

Konstantinov IE, Mejevoi N, Anichkov NM. Nikolai N. Anichkov and His Theory of Atherosclerosis. Tex Heart Inst, J. Exp Med. 2006; 33(4):417-23.

Duff GL, McMillan GC. Pathology of atherosclerosis. Am J Med. 1951 Jul; 11(1):92-108.

Keys A. Atherosclerosis: A problem in newer public health. J Mt Sinai Hosp N Y. 1953 Jul-Aug; 20(2):118.39.

Keys A (ed). Seven Countries: A Multivariate of Death and Coronary Heart Disease. Cambridge, MA:Harvard University Press, 1980.

Keys A. Coronary Heart Disease in Seven Countries. Circulation 41, no. 1 (1970):1-211.

Keys A. Letter: Normal Plasma Cholesterol in a Man Who Eats 5 Eggs a Day. New England Journal of Medicine 325, no.8 (1991):584.

Ravnskov U. The Cholesterol Myths, 101. Published by Pragmatic Press. Published: Oct 21, 2014

Rosenman RH. The questionable roles of the diet and serum cholesterol in the incidence of ischemic heart disease and its 20th century changes. Homeostasis 1993; 34:1-43.

Multiple Risk Factor Intervention Trial. JAMA. 1982 Sep 24; 248(12):1465-77.

Ramsay LE, Yeo WW, Jackson PR. Dietary reduction of serum cholesterol concentration: time to think again. British Medical Journal 1991; 303:953-957.

Shaper AG. Cardiovascular studies in the Samburu tribe of northern Kenya. American Heart Journal 1962; 63:437-442.

Mann GV, Shaffer RD, Sandstead HH. Cardiovascular disease in the Masai. Journal of Atherosclerosis Research 1964; 4:289-312.

Day J, and others. Anthropometric, physiological and biochemical differences between urban and rural Maasai. Atherosclerosis 1976; 23:357-361.

Ganong WF. Factors influencing plasma cholesterol levels. In: Review of medical physiology. Los Altos, CA, USA; 1971:224.

Hunninghake DC, Probstfield JL. Drug treatment of hyperlipoproteinemia in hyperlipidemia. In Hyperlipidemia: Diagnosis and Therapy. BM. Rifkind and RI. Levy, editors. New York, Grune and Stratton, 1977, pp 337-362.

Oliver MF. Consensus or Nonconsensus on coronary heart disease. The Lancet 325, no. 8437(1985):1087-89.

Steinberg D. Thematic review series: the pathogenesis of atherosclerosis. An interpretive history of the cholesterol controversy, part V: the discovery of the statins and the end of the controversy. J. Lipid Res. 2006; 47(7):1339-51.

Moore TJ. The Cholesterol Myth. The-Atlantic, VOL:v264, ISS:n3, DATE: Sept 1989, PAGE:37(25), ISSN: 0276-9077.

Yudkin J. Dietary and coronary thrombosis. Lancet. 2.155-162. 1957.

Castleman B, McNeely BU. Case records of the Massachusetts General Hospital. Weekly clinicopathological exercises. Normal laboratory values. N Engl J Med. 1970 Dec 3; 283(23):1276-85.

Van De Graaff KM, Fox SI. Some laboratory tests of clinical importance. In: Concepts of Human anatomy and physiology. Dubuque, IA, USA; 1995:941.

(NCEP) Report. Circulation 2004; 110:227-239.

Stemmermann GN, Chyou PH, Kagan A, Nomura AM, Jano K. Serum Cholesterol and mortality among Japanese-American men. The Honolulu (Hawaii) Heart Program. Arch Intern Med. 1991 MY; 151(5):969-72.

Winder E, Ewers-Grabow U, Thierry J, Walli A, Seidel D, Greten H. The prognostic value of hypocholesterolemia in hospitalized patients. Clin Investig. 1994 Dec; 72(12):939-43.

National Heart, Lung and Blood Institute, Integrated Guidelines for Cardiovascular Health and Risk Reduction in Children and Adolescents.

Expert panel on integrated guidelines for cardiovascular health and risk reduction in children and adolescents: summary report. Pediatrics December 1, 2011:128(5); S213-S256.

Pediatric Cholesterol Guidelines to Adolescents, Young Adults Would Significantly Increase Use of Statins Among This Age Group. JAMA Pediatrics April 6, 2015.

Zhonghua Yi Xue Za Zhi (Taipei). Serum cholesterol levels and prevalence of hypercholesterolemia in school-aged Taiwanese children and adolescents: the Taichung Study.1999 Nov; 62(11):787-94.

Sitadevi C, Patrudu MB, Kumar YM, Raju GR, Suryaprabha K. Longitudinal study of serum lipids and lipoproteins in normal pregnancy and puerperium. Trop Geogr Med. 1981 Sep; 33(3):219 -23.

Warth MR, Arky RA, Knopp RH. Lipid metabolism in pregnancy. II. Altered lipid composition in intermediage, very low, low and high-density lipoprotein fractions. J Clin Endocrinol Metab. 1975 Oct; 41(4):649-55.

Martin U, Davies C, Hayavi S, Hartland A, Dunne F. Is normal pregnancy atherogenic? Clin Sci (Lond). 1999 Apr; 96(4):421-5.

Smolarczyk R, Romejko E, Wojcicka-Jagodzinska J, Czajkowski K, Teliga-Czajkowska J, Piekarski P. Lipid metabolism in women with threatened abortion. Ginekol Pol. 1996 Oct; 67(10):481-7.

Hochman M, M.D, McCormich D, M.D, M.P.H. Endpoint Selection and Relative (Versus Absolute) Risk Reporting in Published Medication Trials. Gen Intern Med. 2011 Nov; 26(11): 1246–1252.

Safety, life-saving efficacy of statins have been exaggerated, says scientist. Science Daily February 20, 2015.

de Lorgeril M, Salen P, Abramson J, Dodin S, Hamazzaki T, et al. Cholesterol lowering, cardiovascular diseases, and the rosuvastatin-JUPITER controversy: a critical reappraisal. Intern Med. 2010 Jun 28; 170(12):1032-6.

Sukhija, Rishi, Prayaga, Sastry, Marashdeh, et al. Effects of Statins on Fasting Plasma Glucose in Diabetic and Nondiabetic Patients. Journal of Investigative Medicine. March 2009 – Volume 57, Issue 3, pp 495-99.

Goldstein MR, Mascitelli L. Do Statins Cause Diabetes? Current Diabetes Reports June 2013, Volume 13, Issue 3, pp 381-390.

Sattar N, Preiss D, Murray HM, Welsh P, Buckley BM, de Craen AJ, et al. Statins and risk of incident diabetes: a collaborative meta-analysis of randomised statin trials. Lancet. 2010 Feb 27; 375(9716):735-42.

Risk Calculator for Cholesterol Appears Flawed. York Times. Nov 17, 2013.

Robinson JG, M.D., M.P.H., Farnier M, M.D., Ph.D., Krempf M, M.D., Bergeron J, M.D., Luc G, M.D., Averna M, M.D., et al. Efficacy and Safety of Alirocumab in Reducing Lipids and Cardiovascular Events. New England Journal of Medicine, April 16, 2015; 372:1489-99.

Chapter 5

Luckman SP, Hughes DE, Coxon FP, Graham R, Russell G, Rogers MI. Nitrogen-containing bisphosphonates inhibit the mevalonate pathway and prevent post-translation prenylation of GTP-binding proteins, including Ras. J Bone Miner Res. 1998 Apr; 13(4):581-589.

Papapetrou PD. Bisphosphonate-associated adverse events. HORMONES 2009, 8(2):96-110.

Lazarou J, Pomeranza BH, Corey PN. Incident of adverse drug reactions in hospitalized patients: a meta-analysis of prospective studies. Jama 1998 Apr 15; 279(15):1200-5.

James, JT, Ph.D. A New, Evidence-based Estimate of Patient Harms Associated with Hospital Care. Journal of Patient Safety: Sept 2013 – volume 9 – Issue 3 – pp 122-28.

Available at: http://www.fda.gov/Safety/MedWatch/SafetyInformation/SafetyAlertsforHumanMedicalProducts/ucm494252.htm. Accessed April 13th 2016.

Orwoll E, Ettinger M, Weiss S, et al. Alendronate for the treatment of osteoporosis in men. NEJM 2000; 343:604-10.

Dzugan SS, Dzugan SA. The cumulative effect of bisphosphonates and statins on stress fractures. Is it a failure of steroid biosynthesis? Neuroendocrinol Lett (NEL). 2016; 37(2):101-5.

Tully PJ, Debette S, Dartigues JF, Helmer C, Areto S, Tzourio C. Antihypertensive Drug Use, Blood Pressure Variability, and Incident Stroke Risk in Older Adults: Three-City Cohort Study. Stroke. 2016 Mar 24.

Pandit AK, Kumar P, Kumar A, Chakravarty K, Misra, Prasad K. High-dose statin therapy and risk of intracerebral hemorrhage: a meta-analysis. Acta Neurol Scand. 2015 Dec 9.

Erie JC, Pueringer MR, Brue SM, Chamberlain AM, Hodge DO. Use and Incident Cataract Surgery: A Case-Control Study. Opthalmic Epidemiol. 2016 Feb; 23(1):40-5.

Russell RG, Bisphosphonates: The first 40 years. Bone 2011 July; 49(1):2-19.

Ebetina FH, Hogan AM, Sun S, Tsoumpra MK, Duan X, Tiffitt JT, et al. The relationship between the chemistry and biological activity of the bisphosphonate. Bone. 2011 July; 49(1):20-33.

Montgomery CO, Bracey JW, Suva LJ. Bisphosphonates: the good, the bad, and the unidentified. AAOS Now. Dec 2011.

Available at: http://humansarefree.com. Accessed Nov 16 2015. Drugging America: 19 Statistics Almost Too Crazy to Believe.

Available at: http://www.rxlist.com/lipitor-drug/clinical-pharmacology. htm. Accessed Nov 7 2015.

Available at: https://www.crestortouchpoints.com/about-crestor/ pharmacokinetics/. Accessed Nov 7 2015.

Gur A, Cevik R, Sarac AJ, Colpan L, Em S. Hypothalamic-pituitary-gonadal axis and cortisol in young women with primary fibromyalgia: the potential roles of depression, fatigue, and sleep disturbance in the occurrence of hypocortisolism. Ann Rheum Dis. 2004 Nov; 63(11):1504-6.

Young AH, Gallagher P, Porter RJ. Elevation of the cortisol-dehydroepiandrosterone ratio in drug-free depressed patients. Am J Psychiatry. 2002 Jul; 159(7):1237-9.

Marklund N, Peltonen M, Nilsson TK, Olsson T. Low and high circulating cortisol levels predict mortality and cognitive dysfunction early after stroke. J Intern Med. 2004 Jul; 256(1):15-21.

Westergaard GC, Suomi SJ, Chavanne TJ, et al. Physiological correlates of aggression and impulsivity in free-ranging female primates. Neuropsychopharmacology. 2003 Jun; 28(6):1045-55.

Brewer-Smyth K, Burgess AW, Shukts J. Physical and sexual abuse, salivary cortisol, and neurologic correlates of violent criminal behavior in female prison inmates. Biol Psychiatry. 2004 Jan 1; 55(1):21-31.

Trakman-Bendz L, Alling C, Oreland L, et al. Prediction of suicidal behavior from biologic tests. J Clin Psychopharmacol. 1992 Apr; 12(2 Suppl):21S-26S.

van de Wiel, van Goozen SH, Matthys W, et al. Cortisol and treatment effect in children with disruptive behavior disorders: a preliminary study. J Am Acad Child Adolesc Psychiatry. 2004 Aug; 43(8):1011-8.

Backhaus J, Junghanns K, Hohagen F. Sleep disturbances are correlated with decreased morning awakening salivary cortisol. Psychoneuroendocrinology. 2004 Oct; 29(9):1184-91.

Jacobs DR Jr, Iribarren C. Invited commentary: low cholesterol and nonatherosclerotic disease risk: persistently perplexing question. Am J Epidemiol. 2000 Apr 15; 151(8):748-51.

Harris HW, Gosnell JE, Kumwenda Z. The lipemia of sepsis: triglyceride-rich lipoproteins as agents of innate immunity. J Endotoxin Res. 2000; 6(6):421-30.

Wilson RF, Barletta JF, Tyburski JG. Hypocholesterolemia in sepsis and critically ill or injured patients. Crit Care. 2003 Dec; 7(6):413-4.

Dunham CM, Fealk MH, Sever WE 3rd. Following severe injury,

hypocholesterolemia improves with the convalescene but persists with organ failure or onset of infection. Crit Care. 2003 Dec; 7(6):R145-53.

Swaner JC, Connor WE. Hypercholesterolemia of total starvation: its mechanism via tissue mobilization of cholesterol. Am J Physiol. 1975 Aug; 229(2):365-9.

Lehtonen A, Viikari J. Serum lipids in soccer and ice-hockey players. Metabolism.1980 Jan; 29(1):36-9.

Jakovljevic M, Reiner Z, Milicic D. Mental disorders, treatment response, mortality and serum cholesterol: a new holistic look at old data. Psychiatr Danub. 2007 Dec; 19(4):207-81.

Boston PF, Dursun SM, Reveley MA. Cholesterol and mental disorders. Br J Psychiatry. 1996 Dec; 169(6):682-9.

Tierney E, Bukelis I, Thompson RE, Ahmed K, Aneja A, Kratz L, Kelley RI. Abnormalities of cholesterol metabolism in autism. Am J Med Genet B Neuropsychiatr Genet. 2006 Sept 5; 141B(6):666-8.

Golomb BA, Stattin H, Mednick S. Low cholesterol and violent crime. J Psychiatr Res. 2000 Jul-Oct; 34(4-5):301-9.

Forette B, Tortrat D, Wolmark Y. Cholesterol as risk factor for mortality in elderly women. Lancet. 1989 Apr 22; 1(8643):868-70.

Olsen TS, Christensen RH, Kammersgaard LP, Andersen KK. Higher total serum cholesterol levels are associated with less severe strokes and lower all-cause mortality: ten-year follow-up of ischemic strokes in the Copenhagen Stroke Study. Stroke. 2007 Oct; 38(10):2646-51.

Iribarren C, Reed DM, Burchfiel CM, Dwyer JH. Serum total cholesterol and mortality. Confounding factors and risk modification in Japan-American men. JAMA. 1995 Jun 28; 273(24):1926-32.

Neaton JD, Ph.D., Blackburn H, M.D., Jacobs D, Ph.D., Kuller L, M.D., D.P.H., Lee DJ, M.D., Sherwin R, M.B., BChir, et al. Serum Cholesterol Level and Mortality Findings for Men Screened in the Multiple Risk Factor Intervention Trial. Arch Intern Med. 1992; 152(7):1490-1500.

Ladeia AM, Guimaraes AC, Lima JC. The Lipid profile and coronary artery disease. Arq Bras Cardiol. 1994 Aug; 63(2):101-6.

Corti MC, Guralnik JM, Salive ME, Harris T, Ferrucci L, Glynn RJ, et al. Clarifying the direct relation between total cholesterol levels and death from coronary heart disease in older persons. Ann Intern Med. 1997 May 15; 126(10):753-60.

Krumholz HM, Seeman TE, Merrill SS, Mendes de Leon CF, Vaccarino V, Silerman DI, et al. Lack of association between cholesterol and coronary heart disease mortality and morbidity and all-cause mortality in persons older than 70 years. JAMA. 1994 Nov 2; 272(17):1335-40.

Sherwin RW, Wentworth DN, Cutler JA, Hulley SB, Kuller LH, Stamler J. Serum cholesterol levels and cancer mortality in 361,662 men screened for the Multiple Risk Factor Intervention Trail. JAMA 1987 Feb 20; 257(7):943-8.

Stemmermann GN, Chyou PH, Kagan A, Nomura AM, Jano K. Serum cholesterol and mortality among Japanese-American. Honolulu (Hawaii) Heart Program. Arch Intern Med. 1991 May; 151(5):969-72.

Windler E, Ewers-Grabow U, Thierry J, Walli A, Seidel D, Greten H. The prognostic value of hypocholesterolemia in hospitalized. Clin Invstig. 1994 Dec; 72(12):943-8.

Wannamethee G, Shaper AG, Whincup PH, Walker M. Low serum total cholesterol concentrations and mortality in middle aged British men. BMJ. 1995 Aug 12; 311(7002):409-13.

Iribarren C, Reed DM, Chen R, Yano K, Dwyer JH. Low serum cholesterol and mortality. Which is the cause and which is the effect? 1995 Nov 1; 92(9):2396-403.

Sheng R, Chen Y, Yung Gee H, Stec E, Melowic HR, Blatner NR. Cholesterol modulates cell signaling and protein networking by specifically interacting with PDZ domain-containing scaffold proteins. Nat Commun. 2012; 3:1249.

Chapter 6

Available   at:http://www.spacedoc.com/assets/uploads/faers-statin-review_150820_042120_588.jpg. Accessed Nov 15 2015.

Golomb AB, Evans MA. Statin Adverse Effects: A Review of the Literature and Evidence for a Mitochondrial Mechanism. Am J Cardiovasc Drugs. 2008; 8(6):373-418.

Tomlinson B, Chan P, Lan W. How well tolerated are lipid-lowering drugs? Drugs Aging. 2001; 18(9):665-83.

Gaist D, Garcia Rodriguez LA, Huerta C, Hallas J, Sindrup SH. Are users of lipid-lowering drugs at increased risk of peripheral neuropathy? Eur J Clin Parmacol. 2001 Mar; 56(12):931-3.

Gaist D, Jeppesen U, Andersen M, et al. Statins and the risk of polyneuropathy: a case-control study. Neurology 2002 May 14; 58(9):1333-7.

Carvajal A, Macias D, Sàinz M, Ortega S, Martin Arias LH, Velasco A, et al. HMG CoA reductase inhibitors and impotence: two case series from Spanish and French drug monitoring systems. Drug Saf. 2006; 29(2):143-9.

Rizvi K, Hampson JP, Harvey JN. Do lipid-lowering drugs cause erectile dysfunction? A systematic review. Fam Pract. 2002 Feb; 12(1):95-8.

Muldoon MF, Ryan Cm, Flory JD, Manuck SB. Effects of simvastatin on cognitive functioning. Presented at the American Heart Association Scientific Session. Chicago, IL, USA; 2002, Nov. 17-20.

King DS, Wilburn AJ, Wofford MR, Harrell TK, Lindley BJ, Jones DW. Cognitive impairment associated with atorvastatin and simvastatin. Pharmacotherapy. 2003 Dec; 23(112):1663-7.

Orsi A, Sherman O, Woldeselassie Z. Simvastatin-associated memory loss. Parmacotherapy. 2001 Jun; 21(6):767-9.

Wagstaff LR, Mitton MW, Arvik BM, Doraiswamy PM. Statin-associated memory loss: analysis of 60 case reports and review of the literature. Pharmacotherapy. 2003 Jul; 23(7):871-80.

Philllip PS, Haas RH, Bannykh S, et al. Statin-associated myopathy with normal creatine kinase levels. Ann Int Med 2002 Oct 1; 137(7):581-5.

Silver MA, Langsjoen PH, Szabo S, et al. Statin Cardiomyopathy? A potential role for Co-Enzyme Q10 therapy for statin-induced changes in diastolic LV performance: description of a clinical protocol. Biofactors. 2003; 18(1-4):125-7.

Reversal of statin-induced memory dysfunction by co-enzyme Q10: a case report. Health and Risk Management 2015:11 579-581.

Choi HK, Won EK, Choung SY. Effect of Coenzyme Q10 Supplementation in Statin-Treated Obese Rats. Biomol Ther (Seoul). 2016 Mar 1; 24(2):171-7.

Bang CN, Greve AM, La Cour M, Boman K, et al. Effect of Randomized Lipid Lowering With Simvastatin and Ezetimibe on Cataract Development (from the Simvastatin and Ezetimibe in Aortic Stenosis Study). Am J Cardiol. 2015 Dec 15; 116(12):1840-4.

Erie JC, Pueringer MR, Brue SM, Chambelain AM, Hodge DO. Statin Use and Incident Cataract Surgery: A Case-Control Study. Ophthalmic Epidemiol. 2016 Feb; 23(1):40-50.

Holloway V, Wylies K. Sex drive and sexual desire. Curr Opin Psychiatry. 2015 Nov; 28(6):424-9.

Fernandes V, Santos MJ, Pérez A. Statin-related myotoxicity. Endocrinol Nutr. 2016 Mar 19.

Scheen AJ. Fatal rhabdomyolysis caused by cerivastatin. Rev Med Liege. 2001 Aug; 56(8):592-4.

Chang JT, Staffa JA, Parks M, Green L. Rhabdomyolysis with HMG-CoA reductase inhibitors and gemfibrozil combination therapy. Pharmacoepidemiol Drug Saf. 2004 Jul; 13(7):417-26.

Newman TB, Hulley SB. Carcinogenicity of lipid-lowering drugs. JAMA 1996; 275(1):55-60.

William RR, Sorlie PD, Feinleib M, McNamara PM, Kannel WB, Dawber TR. Cancer incidence by levels of cholesterol. JAMA. 1981 Jan 16; 245(3):247-52.

Tornber SA, Carstensen JM, Holm LE. Risk of stomach cancer in association with serum cholesterol and beta-lipoprotein. Acta Oncol. 1998; 27(1):39-42.

Onder G, Landi F, Volpato S, Fellin, Carbonin P, Gambassi G, et al. Serum cholesterol levels and in-hospital mortality in the elderly. Am J Med. 2003 Sep; 115(4):265-71.

Ahmad A, Fletcher MT, Roy TM. Simvastatin-induced lupus-like syndrome. Tenn Med. 2000 Jan; 93(1):21-2.

Wierzbicki AS, Lumb PJ, Semra Y, Chik G, Christ ER, Crook MA. Atorvastatin compared with simvastatin-based therapies in the management of severe familial hyperlipidaemias. QJM. 1999 Jul; 92(7):387-94.

Bakker-Arkema RG, Nawrocki JW, Black DM. Safety profile of atorvastatin-treated patients with low LDL-cholesterol levels. Atherosclerosis. 2000 Mar; 149(1):123-9.

Chung N, Cho SY, Choi DH, Zhu JR, Lee K, Lee PK, et al. STATT: a titrate-to-goal study of simvastatin in Asian patients with coronary heart disease. Simvastatin Treats Asians to Target. Clin Ther. 2001 Jun; 23(6):858-70.

Jacobson TA. Clinical context: current concepts of coronary heart disease management. Am J Med. 2001 Apr 16; 110 Suppl 6A:3S-11S.

Hunninghake D, Insull W, Knopp R, Davidson M, Lohrbauer L, Jones P, et al. Comparison of the efficacy of atorvastatin versus cerivastatin in primary hypercholesterolemia. Am J Cardiol. 2001 Sept 15; 88(6):635-9.

McPherson R, Hanna K, Agro A, Braeken A; Canadian Cerivastatin Study Group. Cerivastatin versus branded pravastatin in the treatment of primary hypercholesterolemia in primary care practice in Canada: a one-year, open-label, randomized, comparative study of efficacy, safety, and cost-effectiveness. Clin Ther. 2001 Sep; 23(9):1492-507.

McKenney JM. New guidelines for managing hypercholesterolemia. J Am Pharm Assoc (Wash). 2001 Jul-Aug; 41(4):596-607.

Simons LA, Levis G, Simons J. Apparent discontinuation rates in patients prescribed lipid-lowering drugs. Med J Aust. 1996 Feb 19; 164(4):208-11.

Lambrecht BN. Immunologists getting nervous: neuropeptide, dendritic cells and T cell activation. Respiratory Research 2: 133-38, 2001.

Pert C. Molecules of Emotion, Scribner, New York, 1997.

Griffithes G, Simons K. The Trans-Golgi Network: Sorting at the Exit Side of the Golgi Complex, Science 243:438-442, 1986.

Golomb BA, Kane T, Dimsdale JE. Severe irritability associated with statin cholesterol-lowering drugs. QJM. 2004 Apr; 97(4):229-35.

Available at: http://www. anma.org/mon62.html. Accessed Dec, 2015.

Go AS, Mozaffarian D, Roger VL, Benjamin EJ, Berry JD, Borden WB, et al. Heart disease and stroke statistics – 2013 update: a report from the American Heart Association. Circulation. 2013 Jan 1; 127(1).

Accessed 30 Dec 2016. http://www.cwru.edu/med/epidbio/mphp439/CongHeartFail.pdf.

Molyneux SL, Florkowski CM, George PM, Pilbrow AP, Framptom CM, Lever M, Richards AM. Coenzyme Q10: an independent predictor of mortality in chronic heart failure. J Am Coll Cardiol. 2008 Oct 28; 52(18):1435-41.

Biochimica et Biophysica Acta (BBA) Moleculare Basis of Disease, Vol 1271, N.1. May, 1995.

Journal of Clinical Pharmacological 33 (3):226-9 dol:10.1002/i.1552-4604. 1993.

Chronic fatigue, aging, mitochondrial function and nutritional supplements. The Townsend Letter, 2003.

Gaist D, Garcia Rodriguez LA, Huerta C, et al. Are users of lipid-lowering drugs at increased risk of peripheral neuropathy? Eur J Clin Pharmacol. 2001 Mar; 56(12):931-3.

Maier O, De Jonge J, Nomden A, Hoekstra D, Baron W. Lovastatin induces the formation of abnormal myelin-like membrane sheets in primary oligodendrocytes. Glia. 2009; 57:402–413.

Saher G, Brugger B, Lappe-Siefke C, Mobius W, Tozawa R, Wehr MC, et al. High cholesterol level is essential for myelin membrane growth. Nat Neurosci. 2005; 8:468-475.

Miron VE, Rajasekharan S, Jarjour AA, Zamvil SS, Kennedy TE, Antel JP. Simvastatin regulates oligodendroglial process dynamics and survival. Glia. 2007; 55:130-143.

Gaist D, Jeppesen U, Andersen M, Garcia Rodriguez LA, Hallas J, Sindrup SH. Statins and risk of polyneuropathy: a case-control study. Neurology. 2002 May 14; 58(9):1333-7.

Wang J, Xiao Y, Luo M, Luo H. Statins for multiple sclerosis. Cochrane Database Syst Rev. 2011 Dec 7; (12).

Miron VE, Rajasekharan S, Jarjour AA, Zamvil SS, Kennedy TE, Antel JP. Simvastatin regulates oligodendroglial process dynamics and survival. Glia. 2007; 55:130-143.

Foote AK, Blakemore WF. Inflammation stimulates remyelination in areas of chronic demyelination. Brain. 2005 Mar; 128(Pt 3):528-39.

Xiang Z, Reeves SA. Simvastatin increases cell death in a mouse cerebellar slice culture (CSC) model of developmental myelination. Exp Neurol 2009 Jan; 215(1);41-47.

Dorst J, Kuhnlein P, Hendrich C, Kassubek J, Sperfeld AD, Ludolph AC. Patients with elevated triglyceride and cholesterol serum levels have a prolonged survival in amyotrophic lateral sclerosis. J Neurol. 2011 Apr; 258(4):613-7.

Dupuis L, Corcia P, Fergani A, Gonzalez De Ajuilar JL, Bonnefont-Rousselot D, et al. Dyslipidemia is a protective factor in amyotrophic lateral sclerosis. Neurology. 2008 Mar 25; 70(13):1004-9.

Golomb BA, Kwon EK, Koperski S, Evans MA. Amyotrophic lateral sclerosis-like conditions in possible association with cholesterol-lowering drugs: an analysis of patient reports to the University of California, San Diego (UCSD) Statin Effects Study. Drug Saf. 2009; 32(8):649-61.

Meske V, Albert F, Richter D, Schwarze J, Ohm TG. Blockade of HMG-CoA reductase activity causes changes in microtubule-stabilizing protein tau via suppression of geranylgeranylpyrophosphate formation: implications for Alzheimer's disease. Eur J Neurosci. 2003 Jan;17(1):93-102.

Huang X, Alonso A, Guo X, Umbach DM, Lichtenstein ML, Ballantyne CM, Mailman RB, Mosley TH, Chen H. Statins, plasma cholesterol, and risk of Parkinson's disease: a prospective study. Disord. 2015 Apr; 30(4):552-9. doi: 10.1002/mds.26152. Epub 2015 Jan 14.

Melville NA. Statin Use Linked to Increased Parkinson's Risk. Medscape. October 26, 2016.

Huang X, Abbott RD, Petrovitch H, Mailman RB, Ross GW. Low LDL cholesterol and increased risk of Parkinson's disease: Prospective results from Honolulu-Asia Aging Study. Mov Disord. 2008 May 15; 23(7):1013-18.

Musumeci O, Naini A, Slonim AE, Skavin N, Hadjigeorgiou GL, Krawiecki N, et al. Familial cerebellar ataxia with muscle coenzyme Q10 deficiency. Neurology 2001; 56:849-855.

Teive HA, Moro A, Moscovich M, Arruda WO, Munhoz RP. Statin-associated cerebellar ataxia. A Brazilian case series. Parkinsonism Relat Disord. 2016 Feb 2.

Klockgether T. Acquired cerebellar ataxias and differential diagnosis. In: Brice A, Pulst SM. Spinocerebellar degenerations. The ataxias and spastic paraplegias. Philadelphia, PA: Butterworth Heinemann Elsevier; 2007:61-77.

Available at: http://www.scielo.br/scielo.php?pid=S0004-282X2012 000200015&script=sci_arttext. Accessed 25 March 2016.

Mathuranath P. Tau and tauopathies. 55(1) 11-16, 2007 Statins and ALS-like Syndrome.

Horwich TB, Hamilton MA, Maclellan WR, Fonarow GC. Low serum total cholesterol is associated with marked increase in mortality in advanced heart failure. Journal of Cardiac Failure 8(4), 2002.

Borrego FJ, Liébana A, Borrego J, Pérez del Barrio P, Gil JM, Garcia Cortés MJ, et al. Rhabdomyolysis and acute renal failure secondary to statins. Nefrologia. 2001 May-Jun; 21(3):309-13.

Ekhart C, de Jong LA, Gross-Martirosyan LD, van Hunsel FP. Muscle rupture associated with statin use. Br J Clin Pharmacol. 2016 Apr 13. doi: 10.111/bcp.12973.

Omar MA, Wilson JP, Cox TS. Rhabdomyolysis and HMG-CoA reductase inhibitors. Ann Pharmacother. 2001 Sep; 35(9):1096-107.

Goldstein MR, Mascitelli L. Do Statins Cause Diabetes? Current Diabetes Reports June 2013, Volume 13, Issue 3, pp 381-390.

Cartagena CM, Ahmed F, Burns MP, Pajoohesh-Ganji A, Pak DT, Faden AI, Rebeck GW. Cortical Injury Increases Cholesterol 24S Hydroxylase (Cyp46) Levels in the Rat Brain. J Neurotrauma. 2008 Sep; 25(9): 1087-1098.

Cederberg H, Stancakova A, Yaluri N, Modi S, Kuusisto J, Laakso M. Increased risk of diabetes with statin treatment is associated with impaired insulin sensitivity and insulin secretion: a 6 year follow-up study of the METSIM cohort. Diabetologia. 2015 May; 58(5):1109-17.

Sultan S, Hynes N. The Ugly Side of Statins. Systemic Appraisal of the Contemporary UnKnown Unknowns. Open Journal of Endocrine and Metabolic Diseases, Vol. 3 No. 3, 2013, pp. 179-185.

Ford I, Blauw GI, Murphy MB, Shepherd J, Cobbe SM, Bollen EL, et al. A Prospective Study of Pravastatin in the Elderly at Risk (PROSPER): Screening Experience and Basel
ine Characteristics. Curr Control Trials Cardiovasc Med. 2002; 3(1): 8.

Strait JB, Lakatta EG. Aging-associated cardiovascular changes and their relationship to heart failure. Heart Fail Clin. 2012 Jan; 8(1):143-164.

Available at: http//www.cdc.gov/nchs/data/databriefs/db177.htm. NCHS Data Brief. No 177, December 2014. Accessed Jan 11, 2016.

Wallach-Kildemoes H, Stovring H, Holme Hansen E, Howse K, Pétursson H. Statin prescribing according to gender, age and indication: what about the benefit-risk balance? J Eval Clin Pract. 2015 Oct 8.

DuBroff RJ. Statin Diabetes Conundrum: Short-term Gain, Long-term Risk or Inconvenient Truth? Evid Based Med. 2015; 20(4):121-123.

Mansi I, Frei CR, Wang CP, Mortensen EM. Statins and New-Onset Diabetes Mellitus and Diabetic Complications: A Retrospective Cohort Study of US Healthy Adults. J Den Intern Med. 2015 Apr 28.

Sukhija, Rishi, Prayaga, Sastry, Marashdeh, et al. Effects of Statins on Fasting Plasma Glucose in Diabetic and Nondiabetic Patients. Journal of Investigative Medicine. March 2009 – Volume 57, Issue 3, pp 495-99.

Maki KC, Ph.D., F.N.L.A., Ridker PM, M.D., M.P.H., Brown WV, M.D., F.N.L.A., Grundy SM, M.D., Ph.D., F.N.L.A., Sattar N, M.D., Ph.D. An assessment by the Statin Diabetes Safety Task Force: 2014 update. Journal of Clinical Lipidology.

Medscape Medical News. Statins Linked to Diabetes and Complications in Healthy Adults Troy Brown, RN. May 22, 2015.

Mansi IA, English J, Zhang S, Mortensen EM, Halm EA. Long-Term Outcomes of Short-Term Statin Use in Healthy Adults: A Retrospective Cohort Study. Drug Saf. 2016 Jun; 39(6):543-59.

Gu Q, Paulose-Ram R, Burt VL, Kit BK. NCHS Data Brief. N. 177, December, 2014. Prescription Cholesterol-lowering Medication Use in Adults Aged 40 and Over: United States, 2003-2012. Available at: www.cdc.gov/nchs/data/databriefs/db177.htm. Accessed Jan 7th 2016.

Goldstein MR, Mascitelli L. Do Statins Cause Diabetes? Current Diabetes Reports June 2013, Volume 13, Issue 3, pp 381-390.

Oliver MF. Cholesterol-lowering and cancer in the prevention of cardiovascular disease. QJM. 2010 Mar; 103(3):202.

Newman, TB. et al. Carcinogenicity of Lipid-Lowering Drugs. JAMA. January 3, 1996-Vol 275, No. 1.

Available at:
http://drsircus.com/medicine/run-from-your-statinrecommending-cardiologist/. Accessed Jan 19, 2016.

Saito A, Saito N, Mol W, Furukawa H, Tsutsumida A, Oyama A, et al. Simvastatin inhibits growth via apoptosis and the induction of cell cycle arrest in human melanoma cells. Melanoma Res. 2008 Apr; 18(2):85-94.

Childs M, Girardot G. Evaluation of acquired data on long-term risk of hypolipidemic treatments. Arch Mal Coeur Vaiss. 1992 Sept; 85 Spec No 2:129-33.

Tomiyama N, Matzno S, Kitada C, Nishiguchi E, Okamura N, Matsuyama K. The possibility of simvastatin as a chemotherapeutic agent for all-trans retinoic acid-resistant promyelocytic leukemia. Biol Pharm Bull. 2008 Mar; 31(3):369-74.

Ormiston T, Wolkowtz OM, Reus VI, Johnson R, Manfredi F. Hormonal changes with cholesterol reduction: a double-blinded pilot study. J Clin Parm ther. 2004 Feb; 29(1):71-3.

Hall SA, Page ST, Travison TG, Montgomery RB, Link CL, McKinlay

JB. Do statins affect androgen levels in men? Results from the Boston area community health survery. Cancer Epidemiol Biomarkers Prev. 2007 Aug; 16(8):1587-94.

Izquierdo D, Foyouzi N, Kwintkiewicz J, Duleba AJ. Mevastatin inhibits ovarian theca-interstitial cell proliferation and steroidogenisis. Fertil Steril. 2004 Oct; 82 Suppl 3:1193-7.

Mastroberardino G, Costa C, Gavelli MS, Vitaliano E, Rossi F, Catalono A, et al. Plasma cortisol and testosterone in hypercholesterolaemia treated with clofibrate and lovastatin. J Int Med Res. 1989 Jul-Aug; 17(4):388-94.

Available at: http://www.cdc.gov/nchs/data/nvsr/nvsr61/nvsr61_04.pdf. Accessed Jan 14, 2016.

Available at: http://www.lipidjournal.com/article/S1933-2874(13)00052-4/abstract. Accessed Jan 14, 2016.

Available at: Why statins have failed to reduce mortality in just about everyone. http://www.lipidjournal.com/article/S1933-2874(13)00052-4/abstract. Accessed Jan 14 2016.

Ridker PM, M.D., Danielson E, M.I.A., Fonseca FAH, M.D., Genest J, M.D., Gotto AM, Jr., M.D., et al., for the JUPITER Study Group. Rosuvastatin to Prevent Vascular Events in Men and Women with Elevated C-Reactive Protein. N Engl J Med 2008; 359:2195-2207 November 20, 2008.

Petretta M, Costanzo P, Perrone-Filardi P, Chiariello M. Impact of gender in primary prevention of coronary heart disease with statin therapy. International Journal of Cardiology. January 7, 2010 Volume 138, Issue 1, pp 25-31.

Available at: http://drsircus.com/medicine/run-from-your-statin-recommending-cardiologist/. Accessed Jan 14, 2016.

McDougall JA, Malone KE, Daling JR, et al. Long-term statin use and risk of ductal and lobular breast cancer among women 55-74 years of age. Cancer Epidemiology, Biomarkers & Prevention; 2013 Sep; 22(9): 1529-1537.

Available at:
http://www.dailymail.co.uk/health/article-2370825/Statins-risk-women-Taking-cholesterol-lowering-drug-years-doubles-chances-common-breast-cancer.html#ixzz3xDrYkihL. Accessed Jan 14, 2016.

Wang A, Stefanick ML, Kapphahn K, Hedlin H, Desai M, Manson JA, Strickler H, Martin L, et al. Relation of statin use with non-melanoma skin cancer: prospective results from the Women's Health Initiative. Br J Cancer. 2016 Feb 2; 114(3):314-20.

Geurian KL. The cholesterol controversy. Ann Pharamcother. 1996 May; 30(5):495-500.

Ravnskov U. Cholesterol lowering trials in coronary heart disease: frequency of citation and outcome. BMJ. 1992 Jul 4; 305(6844):15-9.

Chapter 7

Molecular Transformation of Plant Sources to Progesterone. Cancer Forum Volume 13 No.(5/6), Winter 1994-95.

Fournier A, Berrino F, Clavel-Chapelon F. Unequal risk for breast cancer associated with different hormone replacement therapies: results from the E3N cohort study. Breast Cancer Res Treat.2008 Jan; 107(1):1'3-11.

Chapter 8

Roberts E. Pregnenolone-From Selye to Alzheimer and a Model of the pregnenolone sulfate binging site on the GABA Receptor. Biochemical Pharmacology, Vol. 49, No. 1. pp 1-16, 1995.

Sahelian, R. Pregnenolone, Nature's Feel Good Hormone. Avery Publishing. 1997.

Akwa Y, et al. Neurosteroids: biosynthesis, metabolism, and function of pregnenolone and dehydroepiandrosterone in the brain. Jour Steroid Biochem Mol Biol. 1991; 40(1-3):71-81.
Paul SM, Purady RH. Neuroactive steroids FASEB J. 1992, Mar;6(6):2311-22.

Wu F, et al. Pregnenolone sulfate: a positive allosteric modulator at the N-methyl-D-aspartate receptor. Mol Pharmacol. 1991; 40(3):333-6.

Weng JH, Chung BC. Nongenomic actions of neurosteroid pregnenolone and its metabolites. Steroids. 2016 Jul; 111:54-9.

Roberts E, Fitten LJ. Serum steroid levels in two old men with Alzheimer's disease (AD) before and after oral administration of dehydroepiandrosterone (DHEA). Pregnenolone synthesis may be ratelimiting in aging. In: Kalimi M, Regelson W, editors. The Biological Role of Dehydroepiandrosterone (DHEA). Berlin, de Gruyter, 1990, 43-63.

Mayo W, Le Moal M, Abrous DN. Pregnenolone sulfate and ageing of cognitive functions: behavioral, neurochemical, and morphological investigations. Horm Behav. 2001; 40(2):215-17.

Osuji IJ, Vera-Bolonos E, Carmody TJ, et al. Pregnenolone for cognition and mood in dual diagnosis patients. Psychiatry Res. 2010 Jul 30; 178(2):309-12.

Vallee M, et al. Neurosteroid pregnenolone, dehyrdroepiandrosterone and their sulfate esters on learning and memory in cognitive ageing. Brain Res Rev. 1995; 615(2):267-274.

Darnaudery M, Pallares M, Piazza PV, Le Moal M, Mayo W, et al. The neurosteroid pregnenolone sulfate infused into the medical septum nucleus increased hippocampal aceteylcholine and spatial memory in rats. Brain Res. 2002; 951(2):237-42.

Guth L, et al. Key role for pregnenolone in combination therapy that promotes recovery after spinal cord injury. Proc Natl Acad Sci USA. 1994; 91(25):12308-12.

Steiger A, et al. Neurosteroid pregnenolone induces sleep-EEG changes in man compatible with inverse agonistic GABA receptor modulation. Brain Res. 1993; 615(2):267-274.

Wu F, et al. Pregnenolone sulfate: a positive allosteric modulator at the N-methyl-D-aspartate receptor. Mol Pharmacol. 1991; 40(3):333-6.

George M, et al. CSF neuroactive steroid in affective disorders: pregnenolone, progesterone and DBI. Biol Psychiatry. 1994; 35(10):775-780.

Yeh J, et al. Nicotine and cotinine inhibit rat testes androgen biosynthesis in vitro. J Steroid Biochem. 1989; 33(4A):627-30.

Barbieri R, et al. Cotinine and nicotine inhibit humanfetal adrenal 11,beta-hydoxylase. J Clin Endocrinol Metab 1989; 69:1221-1224.

Dharia S, Parker CR Jr. Adrenal androgens and aging. Semin Reprod Med. 2004 Nov; 22(4):361-8.

Labrie F, Belanger A, Cusan L, Gomez JL, Candas B. Marked decline in serum concentrations of adrenal C19 sex steroid precursors and conjugated androgen metabolites during aging. J Clin Endocrinol Metab. 1997 Aug; 82(8):2396-402.

Belanger A, Candas B, Dupont A, Cusan L, Diamond P, Gomez JL, et al. Changes in serum concentrations of conjugated and unconjugated steroids in 40- to -80-year-old men. J Clin Endocrinol Metab. 1994 Oct; 79(4):1086-90.

Barrette-Connor E, Khaw KT, Yen SS. A prospective study of dehydroepiandrosterone sulfate, mortality, and cardiovascular disease. N. England J Med. 1986 Dec; 315:1519-24.

Watson R, et al. Dehydroepiandrosterone and diseases of aging. Drugs Aging. 1996; 9(4):274-291.

Comstock GW, Gordon GB, Hsing AW. The relationship of serum dehydroepiandrosterone and its sulfate to subsequent cancer of the prostate. Cancer Epidemiol Biomarkers Prev.1993, 2: 3, 219-221.

Stahl F, Schnorr D, Pilz C, Dorner G. Dehydroepiandrosterone levels in patients with prostatic cancer, heart diseases and surgery under stress. Exp Clin Endocrinol. 1992, 99: 68-70.

Voermans C, Condon MS, Bosland MC. Growth inhibition by dehydroepiandrosterone of human prostate cancer cell lines and primary epithelial cultures of rat prostate carcinomas (meeting abstract). Proc Annu Meet Am Assoc Cancer Res. 1996, 37: A1933.

Schmidt PJ, Daly RC, Bloch M, et al. Dehydroepiandrosterone monotherapy in midlife-onset major and minor depression. Arch Gen Psychiatry. 2005; 62:154-162.

De Bruin VM, Vieria MC, Rocha MN, Viana GS. Cortisol and DHEAS plasma levels and their relationship to aging, cognitive function, and dementia. Brain Cogn. 2002; 50(2):316-323.

Haden ST, Glowacki J, Hurwitz S, Rosen C, LeBoff MS. Effects of age on serum dehydroepiandrosterone sulfate, IGF-1, and IL-6 levels in women. Calcif Tissue Int. 2000 Jun; 66(6):414-8.

Labrie F, Diamond P, Cusan L, Gomez JL, Belander A, Candas B. Effects of 12 month dehydroepiandrosterone replacement therapy on bone, vagina, and endometrium in postmenopausal women. J Clin Endocrinol Metab. 1997; 82(10):3498-3505.

Osmanagaoglu MA, Okumus B, Osmanagaoglu T, Bozkaya H. The relationship between serum dehydroepiandrosterone sulfate concentration and bone mineral density, lipids, and hormone replacement therapy in premenopausal and postmenopausal. J Women's Health (Larchmt). 2004 Nov; 13(9):993-9.

Watson R, et al. Dehydroepiandrosterone and diseases of aging. Drugs Aging. 1996; 9(4):274-91.

Yen SS, Morales AJ, Khorram O. Replacement of DHEA in aging men and women. Potential remedial effects. Ann NY Acad Sci. 1995; 774:128-142.

Arlt W, Callies F, Can Clijmen JC, Koehler L, Reinkce M, Bidlingmaier M, et al. Dehydroepiandrosterone replacement in women with adrenal insufficiency. New England Journal of Medicine, 1999; 34(14):1013-20.

Morales AJ, Nolan JJ, Nelson JC, et al. Effects of replacement dose of dehydroepiandrosterone in men and women of advancing age. J Clin Endocrinol Metab 1994; 78:1360-1367.

Buffinton C, et al. Case report amelioration of insulin resistance in diabetes with dehydroepiandrosterone. Amer Jour Med Sci. 1993; 306(5):320-24.

Bates C, Egerman R, Umstot E, et al. DHEA attenuates study-induced declines in insulin sensitivity in postmenopausal women. Ann NY Acad Sci 1995; 774:291-293.

Casson PR, Faquin LC, Stentz FB. Replacement of dehyrdoepiandrosterone enhances T-lymphocyte insulin binding in postmenopausal women. Fertility and Sterility. 1995; 63(5):1027-31.

Casson PR, Andersen RN, Herrod HG, et al. Oral dehydroepiandrosterone in physiologic doses modulates immune function in postmenopausal women. Am J Obstet Gynecol 1993; 169(6):1536-39.

Khorram O, et al. Activation of immune function by hydroepiandrosterone (DHEA) in age-advanced men. Jour Gerontol A Sci Med Sci.1997; 52(1):1-7.

Wolkowitz OM, Reus VI, Roberts E, et al. Antidepressant and cognition-enhancing effects of DHEA in major depression. Ann N Y Acad Sci 1995; 774:337-339.

Villareal DT, Holloszy JO. Effects of DHEA on abdominal fat and insulin action in elderly women and men. JAMA. 2004; 292: 2243-48.

Barrett-Connor E, Ferrara A. Dehydroepian- drosterone, dehydroepiandrosterone sulfate, obesity, waist-hip ratio, and noninsulin-dependent diabetes in postmenopausal women: The Rancho Bernardo Study. J Clin Endocrinol Metab 1996; 81:59-64.

Herrington DM. Dehydroepiandrosterone and coronary atherosclerosis. Ann N Y Acad Sci 1995; 774:271-280.

Gordon GB, Bush DE, Weisman HF. Reduction of atherosclerosis by administration of dehydroepiandrosterone. A study in the hypercholesterolemic New Zealand white rabbit with aortic intimal injury. J Clin Invest 1988; 82:712-720.

Regelson W, Colman C. The Superhormone Promise. New York, Simon & Schuster, 1996.

Loose-Mitchell DS, Stancel GM. Estrogens and progestins. In: Hardman JG, Limbird LE, Gilman AG. Goodman & Gilman's The Pharmacological Basis of Therapeutics, 10th ed. New York, NY: McGraw-Hill; 2001:1597-1635.

Wakatsuki A, et al. Effects of medroxyprogesterone acetate on endothelium-dependent vasodilation in postmenopausal women receiving estrogen. Circulation. 2001; 104: 1773-1778.

Available at:
https://www.ncbi.nlm.nih.gov/books/NBK279050/. Warren MP, M.D., Shu AR, M.D., Dominguez JE, B,A. Menopause and Hormone Replacement. February 25, 2015.

Melton L, et al. Progestins reverse some of the effects of estrogen. TEM. 2000; 11(2):69-71.

Premarin (conjugated estrogen tablet). Wyeath Pharmaceuticals, Inc. 2004; Philadelphia, PA 19101:Full Prescribing Information.

Effects of estrogen or estrogen/progestin regimens on heart disease risk factors in postmenopausal women. Jama.1995; 273199-208.

Pitashny, M.D., Martinez de Morentin H, M.D., Brenner S, M.D. Oral Contraceptives: Their Mode of Action and Dermatologic Applications. Skinmed. 2005; 4(2):101-104, 106.

Edgren RA. Progestogens. In: Givens J, ed. Clinical Use of Steroids. Chicago. Yearbook Medical Publishers; 1980; 1-29.

Oettel M, Mukhopadhyay AK. Progesterone: the forgotten hormone in men? Aging Male. 2004 Sep; 7(3):236-57.

Maggi A, Perez J. Role of Female gonadal hormones in the CNS: clinical and experimental aspects. Life Sci 1985 Sept 9; 37 (10):893-906.

Sanchez MG, Bourque M, Morissette M, Di Paola T. Steroids-dopamine interactions in the pathophysiology and treatment of CNS disorders. CNS Neurosci Ther. 2010 Jun; 16(3):e43-71.

Wei J, Xiao G. The neuroprotective effects of progesterone on traumatic brain injury: current status and future prospects. Acta Pharmacol Sin. 2013 Dec; 34(12): 1485-90.

Sofuoglu M, Mouratidis M, Mooney M. Progesterone improves cognitive performance and attenuates smoking urges in abstinent smokers. Psychoneuroendocrinology. 2011 Jan; 36(1).

Stein DG, Wright DW. Progesterone in the clinical treatment of acute traumatic brain injury. Expert Opin Investig Drugs. 2010 Jul; 19(7):847-57.

Hu Z, Li Y, Fang M, Wai MS, Yew DT. Exogenous progesterone: a potential therapeutic candidate in CNS injury and neurodegeneration. Curr Med Chem. 2009; 16(11):1418-25.

Formby B, Wiley TS. Progesterone inhibits growth and induces apoptosis in breast cancer cells: Inverse effects on Bc1-2 and p53. Ann Clin Lab Sci. 1998; 28(6):360-369.

McDougall JA, Malone KE, Daling JR, Cushing-Haugen KL, Porter PL, Li CI. Long-term statin use and risk of ductal and lobular breast cancer among women 55-74 years of age. Cancer Epidemiol Biomarkers Prev. 2013 Sept; 22(9):1529-1537.

Available at:
http://www.naturalnews.com/041605_statin_drugs_breast_cancer_prostate.html. Accessed March 30 2016

Chang CC, Ho SC, Chiu HF, Yang CY. Statins increase the risk of prostate cancer: a population-based case- control study. Prostate. 2011 Dec; 71(16):1818-24.

Fredricsson K, Carlstrom K, Ploen L. Steroid metabolism and morphologic features of the human testis. Journal of Androlog. 1998 Jan-Feb; 10(1):43-9.

Tesarik J, Mendoza C, Moos J, Carreras A. Selective expression of a progesterone receptor on the human sperm surface. Ferility and Steril. 1992 Oct; 58(4):784-92.

Prior JC. Progesterone as a bone-trophic hormone. Endocr Rev. 1990 May; 11(2):386-98.

Veldscholte J, Voorhorst-Ogink MM, Bolt-de Vries J, van Rooij HC, Trapman J, Mulder E.1990. Unusual Specificity of the Androgen Receptor in the Human Prostate Cancer Cell Line LNCaP: high affinity for progesterone and estrogenic Steroids. Biochim Biophys Acta. 1990 Apr 9; 1052(1):187-94.

Lee JR. 1990. Osteoporosis Reversal. Th Role of Progesterone. Internatinonal Nutrition Review 10(3):384-91.

Rossouw JE, Anderson GL, Prentice RL, LaCroix AZ, Kooperberg C, Stefanick ML, et al. Risks and benefits of estrogen plus progestins in healthy postmenopausal women: principal results From the Women's Health Initiative randomized controlled trial. JAMA. 2002 Jul 17; 288(3):321-33.

Evans J. Horse Breeding and Management: Elsevier; 1992.

Barnes R, Lobo R. Pharmacology of Estrogens. In: Mishell D, Jr, ed. Menopause: Physiology and Pharmacology. Chicago: Year Book Medical Publishers, Inc; 1987.

Khaw KT, Dowsett M, Folk E, Bingham S, Wareham N, Luben R, Welch A, Day N. Endogenous testosterone and mortality due to all causes, cardiovascular disease, and cancer in men: European prospective investigation into cancer in Norfolk (EPIC-Norfolk)

Prospective Population Study. Circulation. 2007 Dec4; 116(23):2694-2701.

Hak AE, Witterman JC, de Jong FH, Greelings MI, Hofman A, Pols HA. Low levels of endogenous androgens increase the risk of atherosclerosis in elderly men: the Rotterdam study. J Clin Endocrinol Metab. 2002 Aug; 87:3632-3639.

Becker KL. Principles and practice of endocrinology and metabolism. 1990, p 786. Lippincott Company. Philadelphia, USA.

Xu X, Roman JM, Issaq HJ, Keefer LK, Veenstra TD, Ziegler RG. Quantitative measurement of endogenous estrogens and estrogen metabolites in human serum by liquid chromatography-tandem mass spectrometry. Anal Chem. 2007; 79:7813-21.

Xu X, Duncan AM, Merz-Demlow BE, Phipps WR, Kurzer MS. Menstrual cycle effects on urinary estrogen metabolites. J Clin Endocrinol Metab. 1999; 84:3914-18.

Helguero LA, Faulds MH, Gustafsson JA, Haldosen LA. Estrogen receptors alpha (ERalpa) and beta (ERbeta) differentially regulate proliferation and apoptosis of the normal murine mammary epithelial cell line HC11. Oncogene. 2005 Oct 6; 24(44):6605-16.

Bardin A, Boulle N, Lazennec G, Vognon F, Pujol P. Loss of ERbeta expression as a common step in estrogen-dependent tumor progression. Endocr Relat Cancer. 2004 Sept; 11(3):537-51.

Isaksson E, Wang H, Sahlin L, von Schoultz B, Masironi B, von Schoultz E, et al. Expression of estrogen receptors (alpha, beta) and insulin-like growth factor-1 in breast tissue from surgically postmenopause cynomolgus macaques after long-term treatment with HRT and tamoxifen. Breast. 2002 Aug; 11(4):295-300.

Weatherman RV, Clegg NJ, Scanlan TS. Differential SERM activation of the oestrogen receptors (ERalpha and ERbeta) at AP-1 sites. Chem Biol. 2001 May; 8(5):427-36.

Pettersson K, Delaunay F, Gustafsson JA. Estrogen receptor beta acts as a dominant regulator of estrogen signaling. Oncogene. 2000 Oct 12; 19(43):4970-8.

Saji S, Jensen EV, Nilsson S, Rylander T, Warner MM, Gustafsson JA. Estrogen receptors alpha and beta in therodent mammary gland. Proc Natl Acad Sci USA. 2000 Jan 4; 97(1):337-42.

Komima T, Lindeim SR, Duffy DM, Vijod MA, Stanczyk FZ. Doses of ethinyl estradiol used in oral contraceptives. Am J Obstet Gynecol. 1993 Dec; 169(6):1540-4.

Colacurci N, Zavone R, Mollo A, Russo G, Passaro M, et al. Effects of hormone replacement therapy on glucose metabolism. Panminerva Med. 1998 Mar; 40(1):18-21.

Wysowski DK. Reports of Esophageal Cancer with Oral Bisphosphonate Use. N Engl J Med 2009; 360:89-90.

Ruggiero SL, Mehrotra B, Rosenburg TJ, Engroff SL. Osteonecrosis of the jaws associated with the use of bisphosphonates: a review of 63 cases. J Oral Maxillofac Surg. 2004; 62:527-534.

Heckbert SR, Li G, Cummings SR, Smith NL, Psaty BM. Use of alendronate and risk of incident atrial fibrillation in women. Arch Intern Med. 2008; 168:826-831.

Miranda J. Osteoporosis drugs increase risk of heart problems. CHEST 2008. Vol Philadelphia, PA: American College of Chest Physicians; 2008.

Compston JE. Sex steroids and bone. Physiol Rev. 2001; 81:419-447.

Miller BE, De Souza MJ, Slade K, Luciano AA. Sublingual administration of micronized estradiol and progesterone, with and without micronized testosterone: effect on biochemical markers of bone metabolism and bone mineral density. Menopause. 2000; 7:318-326.

Villareal DT. Effects of dehydroepiandrosterone on bone mineral density: what implications for therapy? Treat Endocrinol. 2002; 1:349-357.

Jan Kowski CM, Gozansky WS, Kittelson JM, Van Pelt RE, Schwartz RS, Kohrt WM. Increases in bone mineral density in response to oral dehydroepiandrosterone replacement in older adults appears to be mediated by serum estrogens. J Clin Endocrinol Metab. 2008; 93:4767-4773.

LeBlanc ES, Nielson CM, Marshall LM, Lapidus JA, Barrett-Connor E, Ensrud KE, Hoffman AR, et al. Osteoporotic Fractures in Men Study Group. The effects of serum testosterone, estradiol, and sex hormone binding globulin levels on fracture risk in older men. J Clin Endocrinol Metab. 2009 Sep; 94(9):3337-46.

Garnero P, Sornay-Rendu E, Claust B, Delmas PD. Biochemical markers of bone turnover, endogenous hormones and risk of fractures in postmenopausal women: the OFELY study. J Bone MinernRes. 2000; 15:1526-1536.

Massaro D, Massaro GD. Estrogen regulates pulmonary alveolar formation, loss, and regeneration in mice. Am J Physiol Lung Cell Mol Physiol. 2004 Dec; 287(6):L1154-9.

Umar S, Rabinovitch M, Eghbali M. Paradox in Pulmonary Hypertension: current controversies and future perspectives. Am J Respir Crit Care Med. 2012 Jul 15; 186(2):125-31.

Glassberg MK, Choi R, Manzoli V, Shahzeidi S, et al.17β-Estradiol Replacement Reverses Age-Related Lung Disease in Estrogen-Deficient C57BL/6J Mice. Endocrinology. 2014 Feb; 155(2): 441-8.

Available at: https://books.google.it/books?isbn=0684854791. Accessed May 2 2016.

Bassil N, Morley J. Endocrine aspects of healthy brain aging. In Health Brain Aging: Evidence based Methods to Preserve Brain Function and Prevent Dementia, edited by A Desai, 57-74. New Yrk: Elsevier, 2010.

Craig MC, Murphy DG. Estrogen therapy and Alzhiemer's dementia. Ann NY Acad Sci. 2010 Sep; 1205:245-53.

Sherwin B, et al. Estrogen effects on cognition in menopausal women. Neurology. 1997:48(suppl 7):S21-S26.

Ogueta SB, Schwartz SD, Yamashita CK, et al. Invest. Ophthalmol Visual Sci, 1999; 40:1906-11.

Wickham LA, Gao J, Toda I, et al. Acta Ophthalmol Scand, 2000; 78:146-53.

Munaut C, Lambert V, Noël A, et al. Br J Ophthalmol, 2001; 85:877-82.

Nonaka A, Kryu J, Tsujikawa, et al. Invest Ophthalmol Visual Sci, 2000; 41:2689-96.

Boekhoorn SS, Vingerling JR, Uitterlinden AG, Van Meurs JB, van Duijn CM, Pols HA, Hofman A, de Jong PT. Estrogen receptor alpha gene polymorphisms associated with incident aging macula disorder. Invest Ophthalmol Vis Sci. Sci. 2007 Mar; 48(3):1012-17.

Smith W, Mitchell P, Wang JJ. Gender, oestrogen, hormone replacement and age-related macular degeneration: results from the Blue Mountains Eye Study. Aust N Z J Ophthalmol. 1997 May; 25 Suppl 1:S13-5.

Guarneri P, Cascio C, Russo D, et al. Neurosteroids in the retina: neurodegenerative and neuroprotective agents in retinal degeneration. Ann NY Acad Sci. 2003 Dec; 1007:117-28.

Seely EW, Walsh BW, Gerhard MD, Williams GH. Estradiol with or without progesterone and ambulatory blood pressure in postmenopausal women. Hypertension. 1999 May; 33(5):1190-4.

McManus J, McEneny J, Young IS, Thompson W. The effect of various oestrogens and progestogens on the susceptibility of low density lipoproteins to oxidation in vitro. Maturitas. 1996 Oct; 25(2):125-31.

Kampen D, et al. Estrogen and verbal memory in healthy post-menopausal women. Obstet Gynecol. 1994; 83(6):979-983.

Anderson V, et al. Estrogen cognition and woman's risk of Alzheimer's disease. AM J Med. 1997; 103(3A):11S-18S.

Asthana S, et al. Transdermal estrogen improves memory in women with Alzhiemer's disease (abstract). Neurosci Abst. 1996; 22:200.

Kojima T, Lindheim SR, Duffy DM, Vijod MA, Stanczyk FZ, Lobo RA. Insulin sensitivity is decreased in normal women by doses of ethinyl estradiol used in oral contraceptive. Am J Obstet Gynecol. 1993 Dec; 169:1540-4.

Fonseca E, et al. Increased serum levels of growth hormone and insulin-like growth factor (associated with simultaneous decrease of circulating insulin in postmenopausal women receiving hormone replacement therapy). Menopause J North Amer Men Soc. 1999; 61:56-60.

Guicheney P, Leger D, Barrat J, Trevoux R, De Lignieres B, et al. Platelet serotonin content and plasma tryptophan in peri and post-menopausal women: Variations within plasma oestrogen levels and depressive mood.

Bruce A, et al. Estrogens attenuates and corticosterone exacerbates excitotoxin oxidative injury and amyloid beta-peptide toxicity in hippocampus neurons. J Neurochem. 1996; 66(5):1836-1844.

Nike E, et al. Estrogens as antioxidants. Methods Enczymol. 1990; 186:330.

Manonai J, Theppisai U. Effects of oral estriol on urogenital symptoms, vaginal cytology, and plasma hormone levels in postmenopausal women. Jour Med Assoc Thai. 2001; 84:539-544.

Sarrel P, et al. Ovarian hormones: recent findings of cardiological significance. Cardiology in Practice. 1991 Mar-Apr; 14-7.

Sarrel P, Lufkin EG, Oursler MJ, et al. Estrogen actions in arteries, bone and brain. Sci Am Med, 1(44); 1994.

Brawer MK. Testosterone replacement in men with andropause: an overview. Rev Urol. 2004; 6(Suppl 6):S9-S15.

Kazi M, Geraci SA, Kocj CA. Considerations for the diagnosis and treatment of testosterone deficiency in elderly men. Am J Med. 2007; 120(10):853-40.

Salom MG, Jabaloyas JM. Testosterone deficit syndrome and erectile dysfunction. Arch Esp Urol. 2010 Oct; 63(8):668-70.
Moskovic DJ, Araujo AB, Lipshultz LI, et al. The 20-year public health impact and direct cost of testosterone deficiency in US men. J Sex Med. 2013; 10(2):562-9.

Ungureanu MC, Costache II, Preda C, et al. Myths and controversies in hypogonadism treatment of aging males. Rev Med Clin Soc Med Nat Iasi. 2015; 119(2):325-33.

Cawthon PM, Ensrud KE, Laughlin GA, et al. Sex hormones and fragility in older men: the osteoporotic fractures in men (MrOS) study. J Clin Endocrinol Metab. 2009; 94(10):3806-15.

Ransome MI. Could androgens maintain specific domains of mental health in aging men by preserving hippocampal neurogenesis? Neural Regen Res. 2012; 7(28):2227-39.

Sharma R, Oni OA, Gupta K, et al. Normalization of testosterone levels is associated with reduced incidence of myocardial infarction and mortality in men. Eur Heart J. 2015 Oct 21; 36(40):2706-15.

Bassil N, Morley JE. Late-life onset hypogonadism: a review. Clin Geriatr Med. 2010; 26(2):197-222.

Bassil N, Alkaade S, Morley JE. The benefits and risks of testosterone replacement therapy: a review. Ther Clin Risk Manag. 2009; 5(3):427-48.

Andersen P, Norman N, Hjermann I. Reduced fibrinolytic capacity associated with low ratio of serum testosterone to oestradiol in healthy coronary high-risk men. Scand J Haematol 1983; 30(Suppl 39):53-57.

Phillips GB, Pinkernell BH, Jing TY. The association of hypotestosteronemia with coronary artery disease in men. Arterioscler Thromb 1994; 14:701-706.

Wallis CJ, Lo K, Lee Y, Krakowsky Y, Garbens A, Satkunasivam R, Herschorn S, Kodama RT, Cheung P, Narod SA, Nam RK. Survival and cardiovascular events in men treated with testosterone replacement therapy: an intention-to-treat observational cohort study. Lancet Diabetes Endocrinol. 2016 Jun; 4(6):498-506.

Chu L, et al. Bioavailable testosterone is associated with a reduced risk of amnestic mild cognition impairment in older men. Clin Endocrinol 2008; 68(4):589-98.

Cherrier N, et al. Cognitive changes associated with supplementation of testosterone or dihydrotestosterone in mildly hypogonadal men: a preliminary report. J Androl 2003; 24(4):568-76.

Testosterone improves spatial memory in men with Alzheimer's disease and mild cognitive impairment. Neurology 2005; 64(12):2063-8.

Desai AK. Healthy Brain Aging: Evidence Based Methods to Preserve Brain Function and Prevent Dementia. Clin Geriatr Med. 2010 Feb; 26(1).

Okun MS, DeLong MR, Hanfelt J, Gearing M, Levey A. Plasma testosterone levels in Alzheimer and Parkinson disease. Neurology. 2004 Feb 10; 62(3):411-3.

Bialek M, Zaremba P, Borowicz KK, Czuczwar SJ. Neuroprotective role of testosterone levels in the nervous system. Pol J Pharmcol. 2004 Sep-Oct; 56(5):509-18.

Lu PH, Masterman DA, Mulnard R, Cotman C, Miller B, Yaffe K, et al. Effects of testosterone on cognition and mood in male patients with mild Alzheimer disease and healthy elderly men. Arch Neurol. 2006 Feb; 63(2):177-85.Epub 2005 Dec 12.

Henderson VW. Estrogen, cognition and women's risk of Alzheimer's disease. Am J Med. 1997 Sep 22; 103(3A):11S-18S.

Wahjoepramono EJ, Asih PR, Aniwiyanti V, Taddei K, Dhaliwal SS, et al. The Effects of Testosterone Supplementation on Cognitive

Functioning in Older Men. CNS Neurol Disord Drug Targets. 2016; 15(3):337-43.

Morgentaler A, Bruning CO 3rd, DeWolf WC. Occult prostate cancer in men with low serum testosterone levels. JAMA. 1996 Dec 18; 276(23):1904-6.

Schatzl G, Madersbacher S, Haitel A, Gsur A, Preyer M, Haidinger G, et al. Associations of serum testosterone with microvessel density, androgen receptor density and androgen receptor gene polymorphism in prostate cancer. J Urol. 2003 Apr; 169(4):1312-5.

Chodak GW, Vogelzang NJ, Caplan RJ, Soloway M, Smith JA. Independent prognostic factors in patients with metastatic (stage D2) prostate cancer. The Zoladex Study Group. JAMA. 1991 Feb 6; 265(5):618-21.

Vatten LJ, Ursin G, Ross RK, Stanczyk FZ, Lobo RA, Harvei S, et al. Androgens in serum and the risk of prostate cancer: a nested case-control study from the Janus serum bank in Norway. Cancer Epidemiol Biomarkers Prev. 1997 Nov; 6(11):967-9.

Sarosdy MF. Testosterone replacement for hypogonadism after treatment of early prostate cancer with brachytherapy. Cance. 2007 Feb 1; 109(3):536-41.

Pechervsky AV, Mazurov VI, Semiglazov VF, Karpischenko AL, et al. Androgen administration in middle-aged and ageing men: effects of oral testosterone undecanoate on dihydrotestosterone, oestradiol and prostate volume. Int. Androl. 2002. Apr; 25(2):119-25.

Chou TM, Sudhir K, Hutchison SJ, Ko E, Amidon TM, Collins P, Chatterjee K. Testosterone induces dilation of canine coronary conductance and resistance arteries in vivo. Circulation. 1996 Nov 15; 94(10):2614-9.

Lazarou S, Morgentaler A. Hypogonadism in the man with erectile dysfunction: what to look for and when to treat. Curr Urol Rep 2005 Nov; 6(6):476-81.

Yeap BB, Hyde Z, Almeida OP, Norman PE, et al. Lower testosterone levels predict incident stroke and transient ischemic attack in older men. J Clin Endocrinol Metab. 2009 Jul; 94(7):2353-9. doi: 10.1210/jc.2008-2416.

Bolour S, Braunstein G. Testosterone therapy in women: a review. Int J Import Res. 2005 Sep-Oct; 17(5):399-408.

Sarrel P, Whitehead MI. (1985). Sex and menopause: Defining the issues. Maturitas, 7 (3), 217-224.

Rhoden EL, Riberio EP, Teloken C, Souto CA. Diabetes mellitus is associated with subnormal serum levels of free testosterone in men. BJU Int. 2005; 96:867-870.

Stellato RK, Feldman HA, Hamdy O, et al. Testosterone, sex hormone binding globulin and the development of Type2 diabetes in middle age men: respective results from Massachusetts Male Age Study. Diabetes Care, 2000; 23:490-49.

Moller J, et al. Testosterone Treatment of Cardiovascular Diseased Principles and Clinical Experiences. Spring-Verlag, 1984.

Phillips GB, Pinkernell BH, Jing TY. The association of hypotestosteronemia with coronary artery disease in men. Arterioscler Thromb 1994; 14:701-706.

Phillips GB. Relationship between serum sex hormones and the glucose-insulin-lipid defect in men with obesity. Metabolism 1993; 42:116-120.

Barrett-Connor E, von Muhlen DG, Kritz-Siverstein D. Bioavailable testosterone and depressed mood in older men: Rancho Bernardo Study. J Clin Endocrinol Metab: 1999; 84:573-577.

Bland J. Introduction to neuroendocrine disorders. Functional Medicine approaches to Endocrine disturbances of Aging. 2001; Gig Harbor, Washington: The functional medicine institute, 57,71,74.

Fink G, Summner BE, McQueen JK, et al. Sex steroid control of mood, mental state and memory. Clin Exp Pharmacol Physiol. 1998; 25(10):764-775.

Almedia OP. Sex playing with the mind. Effects of oestrogen and testosterone on mood and cognition. Arq Neuropsiauitar. 1999 Sept; 57(3A): 701-6.

Raber J. Detrimental effects of chronic hypothalamic-pituitary-adrenal axis activation. From obesity to memory deficits. Mol Neurobiol 1998; 18(1):1-22.

Schwabe L, Wolf OT. Learning under stress impairs memory formation. Neurobiol Learn Mem.2010 Feb; 93(2):183-8. Epub 2009 Sep 29.

Comijs HC, Gerritsen L, Penninx BW, Bremmer MA, Deeg DJ, Geerlings MI. The association between serum cortisol and cognitive decline in older persons.

Phillips AC, Batty GD, Gale CR, Lord JM, Arlt W, Carrroll D. Major depressive disorder, generalised anxiety disorder, and their comorbidity. Association with cortisol in the Vietnam Experience Study. Psychoneuroendocrinology. 2011 Jun; 36(5):682-90. Epub 2010 Oct 16.

Epel ES, McEwan B, Seeman T, et al. Stress and body shape: stress induced cortisol secretion is consistently greater among woman with central fat. Psychosom Med. 2000 Sep-Oct; 62(5):623-32.

Villareal DT, Holloszy JO. Effect of DHEA on abdominal fat and insulin action in elderly woman and men: randomized controlled trial. JAMA. 2004 Nov 10; 292(18):2243-8.

Black OH, Garbutt LD. Stress, inflammation and cardiovascular disease. J Psychosom Res 2002; 52(1):1-23.

Black PH. The inflammation response is an integral part of the stress response: Implications for atherosclerosis, insulin resistance, type II diabetes and metabolic syndrome X. Brain Behav Immun. 2003; 17(5):350-64.

Yong HA, Gallagher P, Porter RJ. Elevation of cortisol – dehydroepiandrosterone ratio in drug-free depressed patients. Am J Psychiatry. 2002 Jul; 159(7):1237-9.

Goodyer IM, Herbert J, Tamplin A. Psychoendocrine antecedents of persistent first-episode major depression in adolescents: a community-based longitudinal enquiry. Psychol Med. 2003 May; 33(4):601-10.

van Niekerk JK, Huppert FA, Herbert J. Salivary cortisol and DHEA: association with measures of cognition and well-being in normal older men, and effects of three months of DHEA supplementation. Psychoneuroendocrinology. 2001 Aug; 26(6):591-612.

Young AH. Cortisol in mood disorders. Stress. 2004 Dec; 7(4):205-8.

Gur A, Cevik R, Sarac AJ, Colpan L, Em S. Hypothalamic-pituitary-gonadal axis and cortisol in young women with primary fibromyalgia: the potential roles of depression, fatigue, and sleep disturbance in the occurrence of hypocortisolism. Ann Rheum Dis. 2004 Nov; 63(11):1504-6.

Young AH, Gallagher P, Porter RJ. Elevation of the cortisol-dehydroepiandrosterone ratio in drug-free depressed patients. Am J Psychiatry. 2002 Jul; 159(7):1237-9.

Marklund N, Peltonen M, Nilsson TK, Olsson T. Low and high circulating cortisol levels predict mortality and cognitive dysfunction early after stroke. J Intern Med. 2004 Jul; 256(1):15-21.

Westergaard GC, Suomi SJ, Chavanne TJ, et al. Physiological correlates of aggression and impulsivity in free-ranging female primates. Neuropsychopharmacology. 2003 Jun; 28(6):1045-55.

Brewer-Smyth K, Burgess AW, Shukts J. Physical and sexual abuse, salivary cortisol, and neurologic correlates of violent criminal behavior in female prison inmates. Biol Psychiatry. 2004 Jan 1; 55(1):21-31.

Trakman-Bendz L, Alling C, Oreland L, et al. Prediction of suicidal behavior from biologic tests. J Clin Psychopharmacol. 1992 Apr; 12(2 Suppl):21S-26S.

van de Wiel, van Goozen SH, Matthys W, et al. Cortisol and treatment effect in children with disruptive behavior disorders: a preliminary study. J Am Acad Child Adolesc Psychiatry. 2004 Aug; 43(8):1011-8.

Backhaus J, Junghanns K, Hohagen F. Sleep disturbances are correlated with decreased morning awakening salivary cortisol. Psychoneuroendocrinology. 2004 Oct; 29(9):1184-91.

Starkman MN, Gebarski SS, Berent S, Schteingart DE. Hippocampus formation volume, memory dysfunction, and cortisol levels in patients with Cushing's syndrome. Biol Psychiatry. 1992 Nov 1; (32):756-65.

Starkman MN, Giordani B, Gebarski SS, Berent S, Schork MA, Schteingart DE. Decrease in cortisol reverses human hippocampal atrophy following treatment of Cushing's disease. Biol Psychiatry. 1999 Dec 15; 46(12):1595-1602.

Lupien SJ, Maheu F, Tu M, Fiocco A, Schramek TE. The effects of stress and stress hormones on human cognition. Implications for the field of brain and cognition. Brain Congn. 2007 Dec; 65(3):209-37.

Eigh E, Lindqvist Astot A, Fagerlund M, et al. Cognitive dysfunction, hippocampal atrophy and glucocortoid feedback in Alzheimer's disease. Biol Psychiatry.2006 Jan; 15:59(2):155-61.

Nawata H, Yanase T, Goto K, Okabe T, Ashida K. Mechanism of action of anti-aging DHEA-S and the replacement of DHEA-S. Mech Ageing Dev. 2002 Apr 30; 123(8):1101-6.

Zietz B, Hrach S, Scholmerich J, Straub RH. Differential age-related changes of hypothalamus – pituitary – adrenal axis hormones in healthy women and men – role of interleukin 6. Exp Clin Endocrinol Diabetes. 2001; 109(2):93-101.

Ferrari E, Cravello L, Muzzoni B, et al. Age-related changes of the hypothalamic-pituitary-adrenal axis: pathophysiological correlates. Eur J Endocrinol. 2001 Apr; 144(4):319-29.

Cersini G, Morganti S, Rebecchi I, et al. Evaluation of the circadian profiles of serum dehydroepiandrosterone (DHEA), cortisol, and cortisol/DHEA molar ratio after a single oral administration of DHEA in elderly subjects. Metabolism. 2000 Apr; 49(4):548-51.

Noth RH, Mazzaferri EL. Age and the endocrine system. Clin Geriatr Med. 1985 Feb; 1(1):223-50.

Luboshitzky R. Endocrine activity during sleep. J Pediatr Endocrinol Metab. 2000 Jan; 13(1):13-20.

Thorn L, Hucklebridge F, Esgate A. The effect of dawn simulation on the cortisol response to awakening in healthy participants. Psychoneuroendocrinology. 2004 Aug; 29(7):925-30.
Rodenbeck A, Hajak G. Neuroendocrine dysregulation in primary insomnia. Rev Neurol (Paris). 2001 Nov; 157(11 Pt 2):S57-61.

Leproult R, Copinschi G, Buxton O, Van Cauter E. Sleep loss results in an elevation of cortisol levels the next evening. Sleep. 1997 Oct; 20(10):865-70.

Copinschi G. Metabolic and endocrine effects of sleep deprivation. Essent Psychopharmacol. 2005; 6(6):341-7.

Briegel J. Cortisol in critically ill patients with sepsis--physiological functions and therapeutic implications] Wien Klin Wochenschr. 2002; 114 Suppl 1:9-19.

Maurer RA. Relationship between estradiol, ergocryptine, and thyroid hormone: effects on prolactin synthesis and prolactin messenger ribonucleic acid levels. Endocrinology. 1982 May; 110(5):1515-20.

Dr Zahid Naeem MBBS, MCPS, DPH, FCPS, Professor. Vitamin D Deficiency – An Ignored Epidemic Int J Health Sci (Qassim). 2010 Jan; 4(1): V-VI.

Hollick MF, Chen TC. Vitamin D deficiency a worldwide problem with health consequences. Am J Clin Nutr. 2008; 87:10805-68.

Calvo MS, Whiting SJ, Barton CN. Vitamin D intake, A global perspective of current status. J Nutr. 2007; 135:310-7.

Iqbal R, Khan A. Possible causes of vitamin D deficiency. J Pak Med Asso. 2010; 60(1):1-2.

Fernandes de Abreu DA, Eyles D, Féron F. Vitamin D, a neuro-immunomodulator: implications for neurodegenerative and autoimmune diseases. Psychoneuroendocrinology. 2009 Dec; 34 Suppl 1:S265-77.

Chapter 9

Dzugan SA, Smith RA. Hypercholesterolemia treatment: a new hypothesis or just an accident. Med Hypotheses:2002; 59:751-6.
Bachmann GA. Androgen cotherapy in menopause: evolving benefits and challenges. Am J Obstet Gynecol. 1999 Mar; 180(3 Pt2):S308-11.

Regelson W, Loria R, Kalimi M. Hormonal Intervention: "buffer hormones" or "state dependency". The role of dehydroepiandrosterone, thyroid hormone, estrogen and hypophysectomy in aging. Ann NY Acad Sci. 1988; 521:260-73.

Morales AJ, Nolan JJ, Nelson JC, Yen SS. Effects of replacement dose of dehydroepiandrosterone in men and women of advancing age. J Clin Endocrinol Metab. 1994. Jun; 78(6):1360.7.

Takahshi K, Manabe A, Okada M, Kurioka H, Kanasaki H, Miyazaki K. Efficacy and safety of oral estriol for managing postmenopausal symptoms. Maruritas. 2000 Feb 15; 34(2):169-77.

Haddock BL, Marshak HP, Mason JJ, Blix G. The effects of hormone replacement therapy and exercise on cardiovascular disease risk factors in menopausal women. Sports Med. 2000. Jan; 29(1):39-49.

Haug A, Hostmark AT, Spydevold O. Plasma lipoprotein responses to castration and androgen substitution in rats. Metabolism. 1984; 33:465-70.

Hanggi W, Birkhauser MH, Malek A, Penheim E, von Hospenthal JU. Cyclical gestagen (MPA) supplement for continuous transdermal or oral estrogen substitution in postmenopause: modification of serum lipids. Geburtshilfe Frauenheilkd. 1993; 53:709-14.

Dzugan SA, Rozakis GW, Dzugan SS, Smith R. Hormonorestorative therapy is a promising method for hypercholesterolemia treatment. Appraches to Aging Control. 2009; 13:12-9.

Dzugan SA, Rozakis GW, Dzugan KS, Emhof L, Dzugan SS, Xydas C, et al. Correction of Steroidopenia as a New Method of Hypercholesterolemia Treatment. Neuroendocrinol Lett (NEL). 2011; 32(1):77-81.

Mastroberardino G, Costa C, Gavelli MS, Vitaliano E, Rossi F, Catalono A, et al. Plasma cortisol and tesosterone in hypercholesterolemia treated with clofibrate and lovastatin. JInt Med Res. 1989; 17:388-94.

Boizel R, de Peretti E, Cathiard AM, Halimi S, Bost M, Berthezene F, et al. Pattern of plasma levels of cortisol, dehydroepiandrosterone, and pregnenolone sulphate in normal subjects and in patients with homozygous familial hypercholesterolemia during ATCH infusion. Clin Endocrinol. 1986; 25363-71.

Broitman SA, Dietary cholesterol, serum cholesterol, and colon cancer: a review. Adv Exp Med Biol. 1986; 206:137-52.

Epstein FH. Low serum cholesterol, cancer and other noncardiovascular disorders. Atherosclerosis. 1992; 94:1-12.

Freeman ME, Kanyicska B, Lerant A, Nagy G. Prolactin: structure, function, and regulation of secretion. Physiol Rev. 2000 Oct; 80(4):1523-631.

Dzugan SA, Rozakis GW, Dzugan KS, Emhof L, Dzugan SS, Xydas C, et al. Correction of Steroidopenia as a New Method of Hyprercholesterolemia Treatment. Neuroendocrinol Lett (NEL). 2011; 32(1):77-81.

Prasad AS, Mantzoros CS, Beck FW, Hess JW, Brewer GJ. Zinc status and serum testosterone levels of healthy adults. Nutrition. 1996 May; 12(5):344-8.

INDEX

Introductory Note
When the text is within a table, the number span is in italic.
     Eg, cholesterol, aging process *80*-1, 160
When the text is within a figure, the number span is in bold.
     Eg, cardiovascular system 1-4, **2**, 92
Roman numerals indicate introductory material.
     Eg, hormonorestorative therapy xvii, 147-**8**, 153, 159-60, 164
     3-hydroxy-3-methylglutaryl CoA (HMG-CoA) 15, 69–70, 94
     2013 guidelines 44–5, 45–6, 65

hormone homeostasis 109, 114,
    123
hormonodeficit hypothesis
    141–2, 142–3, 143–5, 146–7,
    151, 153–4, 158
restorative medicine 52
restorative vs conventional
    medicine 85, 87, 88, 92
Norum, K. R. 40

ODYSSEY drug study 50
omega-3 fatty acids 19, 25, 160
online risk calculator 48–9
optimal health
definition 92–3
hormonodeficit hypothesis 143,
    154–5, 158–9, 160
metabolism of cholesterol 102,
    107–8, 133–4
restorative medicine 85, 87, 90
optimizing physiology 154–5
OSLER drug study 50
osteoporosis
bisphosphonates 55–6
calcium connection 10
metabolism of cholesterol 108,
    114, 115, 119–20, 126, 140
restorative medicine 89
ovaries
hormonal system **95**, 99, 100–1
steroid hormones 103, 107, 112,
    118, 125, 130
thyroid-adrenal function 138
overuse of pharmaceutical drugs
    57–8, 126
oxidation 16, 29–30, 30–1, 123
oxidized LDL (low-density
    lipoprotein) xv, 3–4, 6, 29–30,
    31, 161

pancreas 4, 95, 100, 101, 134, 139
Parkinson's Disease (PD) 75, 76
PCSK9 (proprotein-convertase-
    subtilisin-kexin-9) inhibitors
    14, 49–50, 51, 150, 153, 154
peripheral nervous system 17, 96
PH (pulmonary hypertension)
    120–1
pharmaceutical drugs 53–5, 57–8,
    89, 131
pharmaceutical industries 14,
    41–2, 50, 57, 91, 148
pharmacological doses 90
physiological demand 58, 61–2,
    137, 164
physiological doses 90
pineal gland 99
pituitary gland 95, 98, 100, 102,
    138–9, 159
plaque build-up 7–9, 33
platelets (thrombocytes) 3, 7–8,
    10, 12–13, 123, 156
pregnancy 44, 59–61, 62, 112, 164
pregnenolone
balanced hormones 99, 103–6,
    114, 122
child development 59–61
hormonodeficit hypothesis
    152–3, 154, 156, 160
pathways of steroid hormones
    19–21
pregnenolone steal 61, 105, 137
Premarin (synthetic estrogen) 92,
    110, 115–16
PremPro (synthetic HRT drug)
    110, 115
prescription drugs 53–5, 57–8,
    89, 131
primary prevention 38, 45, 46,
    79–80, 83